Hysterectomy Matters

Edited by Zouhair O. Amarin

Published in London, United Kingdom

Hysterectomy Matters
http://dx.doi.org/10.5772/intechopen.107630
Edited by Zouhair O. Amarin

Contributors
Petre Bratila, Anca Manta, Alexandra Paun, Elvira Bratila, Mehmet Baki Şentürk, Batuhan Üstün, Çetin Çam, Eman Alshawish, Gatot Purwoto, Kartiwa Hadi Nuryanto, Zouhair O. Amarin, Omar Farouq Al tal, Sharifah Halimah Jaafar, Shahridan Mohd Fathil, Iskandar Khalid

First published in London, United Kingdom, 2023 by IntechOpen
IntechOpen is the global imprint of INTECHOPEN LIMITED, registered in England and Wales, registration number: 11086078, 5 Princes Gate Court, London, SW7 2QJ, United Kingdom

British Library Cataloguing-in-Publication Data
A catalogue record for this book is available from the British Library

Additional hard and PDF copies can be obtained from orders@intechopen.com

Hysterectomy Matters
Edited by Zouhair O. Amarin
p. cm.
Print ISBN 978-1-83768-830-2
Online ISBN 978-1-83768-940-8
eBook (PDF) ISBN 978-1-83768-941-5

For EU product safety concerns:
IN TECH d.o.o., Prolaz Marije Krucifikse Kozulić 3, 51000 Rijeka, Croatia,
info@intechopen.com or visit our website at intechopen.com.

Meet the editor

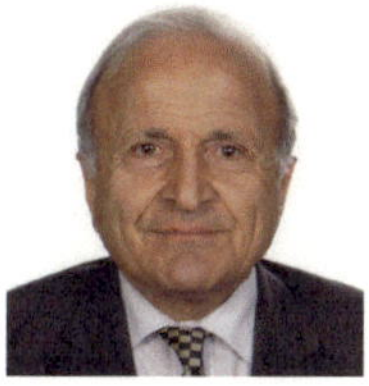

Zouhair Amarin is a Professor of Obstetrics and Gynaecology at the Jordan University of Science and Technology. He was previously a lecturer at the University of Glasgow, Scotland, a senior lecturer at the University of Nottingham, England, and the dean of the Faculty of Medicine at Mutah University, Jordan. Professor Amarin is a fellow of the Royal College of Obstetricians and Gynaecologists, and the Faculty of Public Health, London. He holds master's degrees in medical science and medical education. He is a pioneer in IVF and was the first in the world to develop microsurgical epididymis sperm aspiration for clinical use. He also discovered a surgical procedure for critical ovarian hyperstimulation syndrome. Professor Amarin has edited books, authored book chapters, and published more than 130 papers. He is the recipient of eight awards.

Contents

Preface

Hysterectomy is a common surgical procedure in gynecology. Most women have negative associations with hysterectomy, but the vast majority of those who undergo the procedure do not regret having it performed.

Generally, there has been an observed shift in the type of surgical procedure over time, from abdominal hysterectomy to minimally invasive surgical procedures. Even with the introduction of minimally invasive surgical procedures, hysterectomy is still associated with the risk of intra-operative, immediate post-operative, and short- and long-term complications.

Hysterectomy in younger women may be associated with higher morbidity due to the more active pelvic vascularity. Thus, alternatives to hysterectomy should be considered, especially in cases of dysmenorrhea, dysfunctional uterine bleeding, leiomyomata, endometriosis, or other pelvic health problems.

I would like to thank all the authors for their valuable contributions. I am also grateful to Publishing Process Manager Ms. Ana Javor and the commissioning editors at IntechOpen for their support and advice.

Zouhair O. Amarin
Professor,
Jordan University of Science and Technology,
Irbid, Jordan

Section 1

Hysterectomy Alternatives

Chapter 1

Alternatives to Hysterectomy for Dysfunctional Uterine Bleeding

Zouhair O. Amarin and Omar Farouq Al tal

Abstract

Hysterectomy is a major surgical procedure that is performed through conventional laparotomy, laparoscopy and robotic surgery, or through the vaginal route to avoid abdominal wall incisions. In certain situations, both the abdominal and vaginal routes are used in combination. Hysterectomy is indicated for malignancies of the uterus, uterine cervix, and ovaries; to reduce the risk of future malignancies and genital prolapse; and for dysfunctional uterine bleeding. Dysfunctional uterine bleeding is an aberration caused by hormonal imbalance that is not related to the normal menstrual cycle, with no clear etiology in most cases. Dysfunctional uterine bleeding can be treated medically or surgically. Medical treatment includes non-steroidal anti-inflammatory drugs, the combined oral contraceptive pills, progestogens, danazol, analogs of gonadotrophin-releasing hormone, and the anti-fibrinolytic tranexamic acid. Endometrial ablation and hysterectomy are common routine, low-risk surgical procedures for dysfunctional uterine bleeding but are associated with some comparatively rare serious complications, both operatively and post-operatively. All types of endometrial ablation and hysterectomy remain a mainstay of alternative options for patients where the medical approach proves to be ineffective or is associated with intolerable side effects.

Keywords: hysterectomy, hysterectomy alternatives, dysfunctional uterine bleeding, gynecological drugs, endometrial ablation

1. Introduction

Dysfunctional uterine bleeding is an aberration bleeding that is not related to the normal menstrual cycle. The normal cycle is controlled by hormones that are produced in the right concentration at the right time of the menstrual cycle. Dysfunctional uterine bleeding occurs when the cycle's hormones are imbalanced. In general, no clear etiology can be identified in most cases of dysfunctional uterine bleeding.

In the past, the broad term abnormal uterine bleeding was used to include various etiologies, causing changes in regularity and volume of the bleed, which have been present for 6 months or more, whereas dysfunctional uterine bleeding only covered ovulatory disorders.

Abnormal uterine bleeding, as defined by the Fédération International de Gynécologie et d'Obstétrique (FIGO), in 2011, included polyps, adenomyosis, leiomyomata, malignancy, hyperplasia, coagulopathy, ovulatory, endometrial, iatrogenic, and other unclassified disorders. The acronym PALM-COEIN was used to cover the causes of abnormal uterine bleeding. Bleeding associated with pregnancy was excluded.

Traditionally, various terms were used to describe abnormal uterine bleeding, such as menorrhagia for regular heavy menses, metrorrhagia for irregular menses, polymenorrhea for menses more frequent than every 21 days, and oligomenorrhea for menses that takes place every 35 days or more.

This chapter very briefly outlines hysterectomy and its most common complications, followed by alternatives that may be considered before embarking on this surgical option.

2. Hysterectomy

Hysterectomy is a major procedure that is performed through either the abdominal or vaginal route. Abdominally, the procedure is performed through conventional laparotomy, laparoscopic and robotic surgery. Vaginal hysterectomy avoids abdominal wall incisions. In certain situations, both the abdominal and vaginal routes are used in combination.

Hysterectomy is indicated for malignancies of the uterus, uterine cervix, and ovaries; to reduce the risk of future malignancies as in cases of BRCA mutations; and in Lynch syndrome. In addition, it is indicated for benign conditions that include genital prolapse and for dysfunctional uterine bleeding [1, 2].

Although hysterectomy is a common routine, low-risk surgical procedure, it is associated with some comparatively rare serious complications, both operatively and post-operatively.

3. Hysterectomy complications

The most common complications of hysterectomy may include infection in up to 13% of patients, venous thromboembolism in up to 12% of patients, and genitourinary and gastrointestinal tract injuries in up to 0.6% of patients [3–5].

Blood loss at hysterectomy is about 500 ml; vaginal cuff dehiscence occurs in up to 4% of patients; serious anesthetic complications such as neuropathy, allergy, and death occur in 0.00001% of cases of general anesthesia [3–5].

Hysterectomy may affect the blood supply to the ovaries that may predispose to menopausal symptoms, osteoporosis and ischemic heart disease, lower libido, depression, loss of reproductive capability, negative effect on femininity perception, and a mortality rate of up 1.6 per 1000 hysterectomies [3–5].

In a study that assessed the costs, hospital admission rates, and mortality of 376,246 total hysterectomies, the mortality rates were 0.26%, 0.09%, 0.07%, and 0.05% for supracervical, total abdominal, laparoscopic, and vaginal hysterectomies, respectively [6].

In the same study, total abdominal hysterectomy was financially the costliest of all types, followed by vaginal hysterectomy, supracervical abdominal hysterectomy, and laparoscopic hysterectomy. It was concluded that total abdominal hysterectomy had the highest overall financial cost [6].

4. Alternatives to hysterectomy

Dysfunctional uterine bleeding can be treated medically or surgically. Medical treatment includes non-steroidal anti-inflammatory drugs, the combined oral contraceptive pills, progestogens, the synthetic androgen danazol, analogs of gonadotrophin-releasing hormone (GnRH agonists), and the anti-fibrinolytic tranexamic acid.

5. Non-steroidal anti-inflammatory drugs

Non-steroidal anti-inflammatory drugs reduce the levels of prostaglandins that may be elevated in cases of menorrhagia and dysmenorrhea.

In a metanalysis of nine randomized controled trials, where 759 women were included in the review, prostaglandins were higher in women with heavy menstrual bleeding and were reduced by the administration of non-steroidal anti-inflammatory drugs that were modestly effective compared to tranexamic acid, danazol, and levonorgestrel-releasing intrauterine system (LNG IUS). Those findings were based on a limited number of low- to moderate-quality trials [7].

Similar conclusions were made by a study of published Cochrane Reviews on heavy menstrual bleeding interventions in the Cochrane Database of Systematic Reviews [8].

6. Combined oral contraceptive pills

The combined oral contraceptive pill has various benefits that include the reduction of menstrual blood loss through the regular shedding of a thinner endometrium and the inhibition of ovulation [9].

In a search of the Menstrual Disorders and Subfertility Group trials register for all publications that describe randomized trials of oral contraceptive pills for the treatment of menorrhagia, there was no significant difference in menstrual blood loss between women treated with the oral contraceptive pill and a low dose of danazol, mefanamic acid, or naproxen [9].

A prospective study of 50 women that compared the efficacy and compliance of combined hormonal vaginal ring and oral contraceptive pill in patients with heavy menstrual bleeding suggested that the combined hormonal vaginal ring and oral contraceptive pill are very effective in the short-term therapy for heavy menstrual bleeding [10].

7. Progestogens

Regarding progestogens, a prospective observational cohort study found that medication therapy for women with heavy menstrual bleeding can be successfully implemented at primary care centers, with a low rate of surgery, in conjunction with an improvement in their quality of life [11].

Menorrhagia is a common indication for hysterectomy. Adenomyosis and endometriosis are common causes of menorrhagia and pelvic pain in women of reproductive age; therefore, progestogens could be considered as an alternative to hysterectomy.

In this context, a study aimed at evaluating the effects of etonogestrel implants on pelvic pain and menorrhagia in patients that had not completed their families, thus requiring long-acting reversible contraception and being sufferers from adenomyosis or endometriosis. One hundred women with adenomyosis or endometriosis received etonogestrel implants and were followed-up for 24months. Of these, 74 women completed the 24-month follow-up. There was a significant decrease in pelvic pain and menstrual blood loss [12].

It was concluded that etonogestrel implants were effective in reducing pelvic pain and menstrual flow in women with adenomyosis or endometriosis [12].

8. Danazol

Danazol was synthesized in 1963 and was introduced for medical use in 1971 [13–15]. The mechanism of action of danazol is complex. It acts as a weak androgen, a functional antiestrogen, an anabolic steroid, a weak antigonadotropin, a weak progestogen, and a weak steroidogenesis inhibitor [16–23].

Danazol may be prescribed in cases for endometriosis, fibrocystic breast disease, hereditary angioedema, and other conditions [16–23].

Danazol has been shown to be effective in controlling symptomatic primary menorrhagia [24]. It has to be noted that the use of danazol may be associated with some unacceptable masculinizing side effects such as acne, excessive hair growth, breast atrophy, hot flashes, voice deepening, mood changes, and other long-term side effects [17, 25].

9. Gonadotrophin-releasing hormone analogs

The analogs of gonadotrophin-releasing hormone could be utilized as one of the approaches for the medical management of dysfunctional uterine bleeding. Gonadotrophin-releasing hormone modulators exert their action through their effect on the secretion of the gonadotropins, follicle-stimulating hormone and luteinizing hormone [26–32].

This action, in turn, suppresses the function of the ovaries and their hormone production of sex steroids, including that of estrogen and progesterone, with subsequent endometrial atrophy and improvement of hemoglobin levels [26–32].

Add-back therapy may be considered in cases of long-term use of gonadotrophin-releasing hormone analogs to prevent adverse effects on bone density and vasomotor symptoms without nullifying gonadotrophin-releasing hormone analogs' therapeutic effect.

A combination of both estrogen and progestin or progestin only have been prescribed as add-back therapy with gonadotrophin-releasing hormone analogs. Norethindrone acetate has been used as add-back therapy, as this unique progestin has both estrogenic and androgenic properties, that have been shown to be effective in reducing gonadotrophin-releasing hormone analogs' side effects [33, 34].

10. The anti-fibrinolytic tranexamic acid

The anti-fibrinolytic tranexamic acid exerts its effect by blocking lysine binding sites on plasminogen. This prevents plasmin from acting with lysine residues that affects the fibrin polymer, thus resulting in fibrin degradation in a reversible manner.

In a review that focused on the efficacy and safety of tranexamic acid in the treatment of idiopathic heavy menstrual bleeding, it was found that tranexamic acid was an effective therapy for heavy menstrual bleeding. It reduced menstrual blood loss by up to 60%, being significantly more effective than placebo, nonsteroidal anti-inflammatory drugs, oral cyclical luteal phase progestins, or oral etamsylate [35].

Adverse effects of tranexamic acid are infrequent, with no evidence of an increase in thrombotic events that are related to its use [35].

An active thromboembolic disease or a history of thrombosis or thromboembolism or thrombophilia are considered contraindications for its use [35].

11. Levonorgestrel-releasing intrauterine system

Regarding the utility of the levonorgestrel-releasing intrauterine system in the treatment of dysfunctional uterine bleeding and dysmenorrhea, a thorough and critical overview of previously published research found that that the insertion of a levonorgestrel-releasing intrauterine system was an effective modality in the long term [36].

The original idea for the insertion of a progestogen-releasing device inside the uterus was to utilize it as a long-term contraceptive method. The early devices were associated with unacceptable rates of ectopic pregnancies in cases of contraception failure. On the other hand, it was soon discovered that the system had other useful therapeutic applications, especially for the non-surgical treatment of dysfunctional uterine bleeding [36–39].

Furthermore, levonorgestrel-releasing intrauterine system (LNG-IUS) use in dysfunctional uterine bleeding and dysmenorrhea improves the quality of life, not only by the reduction of menstrual blood loss better than other medical therapies but also by reducing the extent of dysmenorrhea and pelvic pain. In addition, another benefit for some patients is the fact that the system is able to induce amenorrhea, thus eliminating heavy menstrual bleeding and associated dysmenorrhea in women of all ages, especially when contraception is required [39–42].

The levonorgestrel-releasing intrauterine system may be prescribed for anticoagulated patients presenting with dysfunctional uterine bleeding. This approach is associated with a significant reduction in blood loss and an increase in hemoglobin level after less than 6 months of therapy [43].

It has to be noted that with the use of the levonorgestrel-releasing intrauterine system to treat dysfunctional uterine bleeding in patients on anticoagulants, some may experience no improvement, or even experience worsening of their original heavy menstrual blood loss to an unacceptable degree [44].

Glanzmann thrombasthenia is a rare, inherited blood coagulation disorder characterized by defects in the platelet membrane glycoproteins IIb/IIIA. Symptoms of this disorder usually include abnormal bleeding, which may be severe. Female patients with this condition are often troubled with heavy menstrual bleeding [45].

Some adolescents with Glanzmann thrombasthenia have issues with heavy menstrual bleeding beginning at menarche. In a report by Lu and Yang, levonorgestrel-releasing intrauterine system for treatment of heavy menstrual bleeding in adolescents with Glanzmann's thrombasthenia was shown to be associated with a significant reduction of menstrual blood loss along with an improved quality of life [45].

Levonorgestrel-releasing intrauterine system is a potential alternative to other modalities that include anti-fibrinolytics, nonsteroidal anti-inflammatory drugs, and hormonal therapies that are effective, but could be associated with poor compliance.

12. Endometrial ablation

Endometrial ablation is a minimally invasive surgical procedure for the treatment of the common problem of heavy menstrual bleeding. In general, menstruation totaling over 80 ml is considered heavy or excessive.

Several endometrial ablation devices have been approved for women with heavy menstrual bleeding due to benign causes provided that childbearing is complete.

Endometrial ablation device methodology includes heat energy created by heated gas, radiofrequency, free-flowing heated saline that circulates within the endometrial cavity, microwave energy, heated fluid within a balloon, heated water vapor that circulates within the uterus, and extreme cold treatment by nitrous oxide within balloons. All these devices are manipulated into the uterus using an appropriate hand piece.

Potential benefits of endometrial ablation include reduction in menstrual bleeding and improvement in the quality of life. On the other hand, side effects include cramping pain, vaginal discharge, bleeding, and spotting [46].

Late complications following endometrial ablation include post-ablation tubal sterilization syndrome and hematometra due to cervical stenosis [46].

Endometrial ablation does not protect women from future pregnancies. Pregnancy following ablation is hazardous for both the mother and fetus. Sterilization or contraception until menopause should be used. In addition, there may be future difficulty in diagnosing endometrial cancer due to the scarring of the endometrial cavity. Amenorrhea following treatment is not unusual [46].

Endometrial ablation is a more conservative alternative to all types of hysterectomy for dysfunctional uterine bleeding. It is less demanding financially and is associated with shorter hospital stay, but the original indication for its performance is not always resolved. Studies suggest that up to 25% of women undergoing endometrial ablation require further attention, in the form of medications, repeat ablation, or hysterectomy for unacceptable degrees of dysfunctional uterine bleeding [46].

Non-hormonal medications with or without hormonal therapy should be considered before trying more invasive treatments such as endometrial ablation or hysterectomy. Both the American College of Obstetricians and Gynecologists and the National Institute for Health and Care Excellence in the United Kingdom recommend medical therapy for the initial treatment of patients with excessive menstrual blood loss [47, 48].

Endometrial ablation modalities are now a second-line treatment choice after attempting medical therapy that fails for any reason, with the availability of a wide range of well-tested effective devices in use that directly deliver energy to the uterine endometrium. These modalities have demonstrated high levels of success with minimal complications when applied to appropriately selected patients [49, 50].

Hysterectomy remains a definitive surgical modality for patients with dysfunctional uterine bleeding. All types of hysterectomy are considered a mainstay of alternative options for patients where the medical approach proves to be ineffective or is associated with intolerable side effects [51].

Author details

Zouhair O. Amarin* and Omar Farouq Al tal
Jordan University of Science and Technology, Irbid, Jordan

*Address all correspondence to: zoamarin@hotmail.com

References

[1] Chen BH, Giudice LC. Dysfunctional uterine bleeding. The Western Journal of Medicine. 1998;**169**(5):280-284

[2] Jones HW III. Abdominal hysterectomy. In: Rock J, Jones H III, editors. TeLinde's Operative Gynecology. 10th ed. Lippincott Williams & Wilkins, Wolters Kluwer Health; 2008. pp. 727-744

[3] Dicker RC, Greenspan JR, Strauss LT, et al. Complications of abdominal and vaginal hysterectomy among women of reproductive age in the United States. The collaborative review of sterilization. American Journal of Obstetrics and Gynecology. 1982;**144**(7):841-848. DOI: 10.1016/0002-9378(82)90362-3

[4] McPherson K, Metcalfe MA, Herbert A, Maresh M, Casbard A, Hargreaves J, et al. Severe complications of hysterectomy: The VALUE study. BJOG: An International Journal of Obstetrics and Gynaecology. 2004;**111**(7):688-694. DOI: 10.1111/j.1471-0528.2004.00174.x

[5] Wingo PA, Huezo CM, Rubin GL, Ory HW, Peterson HB. The mortality risk associated with hysterectomy. American Journal of Obstetrics and Gynecology. 1985;**152**(7 Pt 1):803-808. DOI: 10.1016/s0002-9378(85)80067-3

[6] Augusto KL, Brilhante AVM, Modesto GCD, Saboia DM, Rocha CFC, Karbage SAL, et al. Costs and mortality rates of surgical approaches to hysterectomy in Brazil. Revista de Saúde Pública. 2018;**52**:25. DOI: 10.11606/S1518-8787.2018052000129

[7] Bofill Rodriguez M, Lethaby A, Farquhar C. Non-steroidal anti-inflammatory drugs for heavy menstrual bleeding. Cochrane Database of Systematic Reviews. 2019;**9**(9):CD000400. DOI: 10.1002/14651858.CD000400.pub4

[8] Bofill Rodriguez M, Dias S, Jordan V, Lethaby A, Lensen SF, Wise MR, et al. Interventions for heavy menstrual bleeding; overview of Cochrane reviews and network meta-analysis. Cochrane Database of Systematic Reviews. 2022;**5**(5):CD013180. DOI: 10.1002/14651858.CD013180.pub2

[9] Farquhar C, Brown J. Oral contraceptive pill for heavy menstrual bleeding. Cochrane Database of Systematic Reviews. 2009;**4**:CD000154. DOI: 10.1002/14651858.CD000154.pub2

[10] Dahiya P, Dalal M, Yadav A, Dahiya K, Jain S, Silan V. Efficacy of combined hormonal vaginal ring in comparison to combined hormonal pills in heavy menstrual bleeding. European Journal of Obstetrics, Gynecology, and Reproductive Biology. 2016;**203**:147-151. DOI: 10.1016/j.ejogrb.2016.05.009

[11] Kai J, Dutton B, Vinogradova Y, Hilken N, Gupta J, Daniels J. Medical treatment for heavy menstrual bleeding in primary care: 10-year data from the ECLIPSE trial. The British Journal of General Practice. 2022;**72**(725):e857-e864. DOI: 10.3399/bjgp.2022.0260

[12] Niu X, Luo Q, Wang C, Zhu L, Huang L. Effects of etonogestrel implants on pelvic pain and menstrual flow in women suffering from adenomyosis or endometriosis: Results from a prospective, observational study. Medicine (Baltimore). 2021;**100**(6):e24597. DOI: 10.1097/MD.0000000000024597

[13] Singh H, Kapoor VK, Paul D. Heterosteroids and drug research. Progress in Medicinal Chemistry. 1979;**16**:35-149. DOI: 10.1016/s0079-6468(08)70187-5. ISBN: 9780720406672. pp. 126, note 158, 130, notes 1513, 2369, citing

[14] Neumann HC, Potts GO, Ryan WT, Stonner FW. Steroidal heterocycles. 13. 4alpha,5-epoxy-5alpha-androst-2-eno[2,3-d]isoxazoles and related compounds. Journal of Medicinal Chemistry. 1970;**13**(5):948-951. DOI: 10.1021/jm00299a034

[15] Elias AN, Gwinup G. Hirsutism. Praeger; 1983. p. 70. ISBN: 9780030603211

[16] Dmowski WP, Scholer HF, Mahesh VB, Greenblatt RB. Danazol--a synthetic steroid derivative with interesting physiologic properties. Fertility and Sterility. 1971;**22**(1):9-18. DOI: 10.1016/S0015-0282(16)37981-X

[17] Danazol Capsules, USP (PDF). Sanofi-Aventis U.S. LLC. U.S. Food and Drug Administration

[18] Brayfield A, editor. Danazol. Martindale: The Complete Drug Reference. Pharmaceutical Press; 2013 [Accessed: April 1, 2014]

[19] Elks J. The Dictionary of Drugs: Chemical Data: Chemical Data, Structures and Bibliographies. Springer; 2014. p. 345. ISBN: 978-1-4757-2085-3

[20] Index Nominum 2000: International Drug Directory. Taylor & Francis; 2000. p. 293. ISBN: 978-3-88763-075-1

[21] Morton IK, Hall JM. Concise Dictionary of Pharmacological Agents: Properties and Synonyms. Springer Science & Business Media; 2012. p. 91. ISBN: 978-94-011-4439-1

[22] Thomas EJ, Rock J. Modern Approaches to Endometriosis. Springer Science & Business Media; 2012. pp. 239-256. ISBN: 978-94-011-3864-2

[23] Jones HW, Rock JA. Te Linde's Operative Gynecology. Walters Kluwer; 2015. pp. 1327-1330. ISBN: 978-1-4963-1521-2

[24] Beaumont H, Augood C, Duckitt K, Lethaby A. Danazol for heavy menstrual bleeding. Cochrane Database of Systematic Reviews. 2002;**2**:CD001017. DOI: 10.1002/14651858.CD001017. Update in: Cochrane Database Syst Rev. 2007;(3):CD001017

[25] Selak V, Farquhar C, Prentice A, Singla A (2007). Farquhar C (ed.). "Danazol for pelvic pain associated with endometriosis". The Cochrane Database of Systematic Reviews. 4: CD000068. DOI: 10.1002/14651858.CD000068.pub2

[26] Colacurci N, De Placido G, Mollo A, Perino A, Cittadini E. Short-term use of Goserelin depot in the treatment of dysfunctional uterine bleeding. Clinical and Experimental Obstetrics & Gynecology. 1995;**22**:212-219

[27] Cetin NN, Karabacak O, Korucuoglu U, Karabacak N. Gonadotropin-releasing hormone analog combined with a low-dose oral contraceptive to treat heavy menstrual bleeding. International Journal of Gynecology & Obstetrics. 2009;**104**:236-239

[28] Khurana C, Taylor P, de Belder MA. Corona stenting in a patient menorrhagia: Use of a gonadotrophin releasing hormone agonist to facilitate anticoagulation. International Journal of Cardiology. 1998;**63**:89-91

[29] Giustozzi M, Vedovati MC, Agnelli G. Management of heavy

menstrual bleeding during direct oral anticoagulant therapy for recurrent venous thromboembolism: A case report. Blood Coagulation & Fibrinolysis. 2018;**29**:391-394

[30] Nencioni T, Penotti M, Barbieri-Carones M, Ortolani S, Trevisan C, Polvani F. Gonadotropin releasing hormone agonist therapy and its effect on bone mass. Gynecological Endocrinology. 1991;**5**:49-56

[31] Thomas EJ, Okuda KJ, Thomas NM. The combination of a depot gonadotrophin releasing hormone agonist and cyclical hormone replacement therapy for dysfunctional uterine bleeding. British Journal of Obstetrics and Gynaecology. 1991;**98**:1155-1159

[32] Thomas EJ. Add-back therapy for long-term use in dysfunctional uterine bleeding and uterine fibroids. British Journal of Obstetrics and Gynaecology. 1996;**103**(Suppl 14):18-21

[33] Adashi EY. Long-term gonadotropin-releasing hormone agonist therapy: The evolving issue of steroidal "add-back" paradigms. The Keio Journal of Medicine. 1995;**44**:124-132

[34] Chwalisz K, Surrey E, Stanczyk FZ. The hormonal profile of norethindrone acetate: Rationale for add-back therapy with gonadotropin-releasing hormone agonists in women with endometriosis. Reproductive Sciences. 2012;**19**:563-571

[35] Leminen H, Hurskainen R. Tranexamic acid for the treatment of heavy menstrual bleeding: efficacy and safety. International Journal of Women's Health. 2012;**4**:413-421. DOI: 10.2147/IJWH.S13840. Epub 2012 Aug 17

[36] Bianchi P, Guo SW, Habiba M, Benagiano G. Utility of the levonorgestrel-releasing intrauterine system in the treatment of abnormal uterine bleeding and dysmenorrhea: A narrative review. Journal of Clinical Medicine. 2022;**11**(19):5836. DOI: 10.3390/jcm11195836

[37] American College of Obstetricians and Gynecologists. Management of abnormal uterine bleeding associated with ovulatory dysfunction. Obstetrics and Gynecology. 2013;**122**:176-185

[38] Matteson KA, Rahn DD, Wheeler TL 2nd, Casiano EA, Siddiqui NY, Harvie HS, et al. Society of gynecologic surgeons systematic review group. Nonsurgical management of heavy menstrual bleeding: A systematic review. Obstetrics & Gynecology. 2013;**121**:632-643

[39] Munro M, Critchley H, Fraser I. Research and clinical management for women with abnormal uterine bleeding in the reproductive years: More than PALM-COEIN. BJOG: An International Journal of Obstetrics & Gynaecology. 2017;**124**:185-189

[40] Heikinheimo O, Fraser I. The current status of hormonal therapies for heavy menstrual bleeding. Best Practice & Research Clinical Obstetrics & Gynaecology. 2017;**40**:111-120

[41] Davies J, Kadir RA. Heavy menstrual bleeding: An update on management. Thrombosis Research. 2017;**151**(Suppl. 1):S70-S77

[42] Rodriguez MB, Lethaby A, Jordan V. Progestogen-releasing intrauterine systems for heavy menstrual bleeding. Cochrane Database of Systematic Reviews. 2020;**6**:CD002126

[43] Kilic S, Yuksel B, Doganay M, Bardakci H, Akinsu F, Uzunlar O, et al. The effect of levonorgestrel-releasing

intrauterine device on menorrhagia in women taking anticoagulant medication after cardiac valve replacement. Contraception. 2009;**80**:152-157

[44] Pisoni CN, Cuadrado MJ, Khamashta MA, Hunt BJ. Treatment of menorrhagia associated with oral anticoagulation: Efficacy and safety of the levonorgestrel releasing intrauterine device (Mirena coil). Lupus. 2006;**15**:877-880

[45] Lu M, Yang X. Levonorgestrel-releasing intrauterine system for treatment of heavy menstrual bleeding in adolescents with Glanzmann's Thrombasthenia: Illustrated case series. BMC Women's Health. 2018;**18**(1):45. DOI: 10.1186/s12905-018-0533-0

[46] Weber AM, Munro MG. Endometrial ablation versus hysterectomy: STOP-DUB. Medscape Women's Health. 1998;**3**(3):3

[47] American College of Obstetricians and Gynecologists. Endometrial ablation: ACOG practice bulletin no. 81. Obstetrics and Gynecology. 2007;**109**:1233-1248

[48] American College of Obstetricians and Gynecologists. ACOG Practice Bulletin No. 110: Noncontraceptive uses of hormonal contraceptives. Obstetrics and Gynecology. 2010;**115**(1):206-218

[49] El-Nashar SA, Hopkins MR, Creedon DJ, Sauver JLS, Weaver AL, McGree ME, et al. Prediction of treatment outcomes after global endometrial ablation. Obstetrics and Gynecology. 2009;**113**(1):97

[50] Lethaby A, Hickey M, Garry R, Penninx J. Endometrial resection/ablation techniques for heavy menstrual bleeding. Cochrane Database of Systematic Reviews (John Wiley & Sons, Ltd). 7 Oct 2009;**4**:CD001501. DOI: 10.1002/14651858.CD001501.pub3. Update in: Cochrane Database of Systematic Reviews. 2013;**8**:CD001501. PMID: 19821278

[51] Reich H, Ribeiro SC, Vidali A. Hysterectomy as treatment for dysfunctional uterine bleeding. Baillière's Best Practice & Research. Clinical Obstetrics & Gynaecology. 1999;**13**(2):251-269. DOI: 10.1053/beog.1999.0021

Section 2

"Morbid" Hysterectomy

Chapter 2

Peripartum Hysterectomy

Mehmet Baki Şentürk, Çetin Çam and Batuhan Üstün

Abstract

Peripartum hysterectomy is a lifesaving surgical procedure that is performed during or immediately after childbirth. Although it is a rare event, it is associated with significant maternal morbidity and mortality. This chapter provides a comprehensive overview of the indications, techniques, and outcomes of peripartum hysterectomy. It also discusses the risk factors, prevention strategies, and management of complications associated with this procedure. The chapter is a valuable resource for obstetricians, gynecologists, and other healthcare professionals involved in the care of pregnant women. It provides evidence-based recommendations and practical guidance to help improve the outcomes of peripartum hysterectomy and ultimately save lives.

Keywords: peripartum hysterectomy, obstetric hemorrhage, cesarean hysterectomy, abnormal placentation, "near-miss" patients

1. Introduction

Life-threatening hemorrhage during or immediately after abdominal or vaginal deliveries is the major cause of maternal morbidity and mortality [1]. Different medical and surgical interventions have been developed to control the hemorrhage, but unfortunately, the removal of the corpus uteri alone or with the cervix at the time of a cesarean section or within the puerperium may be needed as a last resort in saving a woman's life [2]. This procedure is called *peripartum hysterectomy* (PH). On the other hand, if the procedure is performed at cesarean section, it is referred to as *cesarean hysterectomy*, while after vaginal birth, it is called as *postpartum hysterectomy*.

Although the operation may occur as a planned procedure, it is mostly performed in emergency situations to control life-threatening hemorrhage as a lifesaving procedure [3]. Massive hemorrhage and the need to perform the surgery expeditiously create unsuitable conditions both for the surgeon and for women [1].

2. History

Peripartum hysterectomy was first proposed by Joseph Cavallini in 1768 for use in animal models. In 1823, James Blundell demonstrated the feasibility of the idea through experiments conducted on rabbits. Although the method was attempted in humans in 1869, unfortunately, the patient succumbed at the 68th hour following the surgery performed by Storer [4, 5].

The first cesarean hysterectomy in which both the mother and the baby survived was performed by Eduardo Porro from Milan in 1876. During the surgery, Porro passed a wire through the cervix, sufficiently tightening it to control bleeding. He then cut the uterus from above and sutured the stump with silver sutures. As a result, the first human to successfully undergo a cesarean hysterectomy and survive was Julia Cavallini, a 25-year-old dwarf measuring 144 cm in height [1, 4, 5].

Subsequently, the method underwent further modifications by numerous surgeons worldwide.

3. Incidence

The prevalence of PH is reported more frequently in low-resource countries compared to developed countries. In a systematic review and meta-analysis, the estimated overall weighted mean prevalence was reported as 0.9 per 1000 deliveries. Prevalence ranged from 0.2 in some Scandinavian countries to 10.1 per 1000 deliveries in India [6]. Possible reasons for these observed variations are listed in **Table 1** [6, 7].

Additionally, PH is more performed after cesarean section compared to vaginal deliveries [8]. The higher PH rates associated with cesarean sections can be attributed to a higher occurrence of abnormally invasive placentation in these women [1].

If we focus on factors influencing the incidences of peripartum hysterectomies, a strong correlation was observed between the national cesarean section rate and the prevalence of peripartum hysterectomy [9]. Hospitals with high delivery volumes and high rates of hysterectomies saw the largest increases in peripartum hysterectomy rates [10].

Overall, the prevalence or incidence of peripartum hysterectomy is influenced by various factors such as the rate of cesarean section, previous cesarean section, and hospital delivery volume.

4. Indications and risk factors

In a systematic review and meta-analysis, the overall mean maternal age ranged from 26.2 to 37.9 years, the weighted mean gestational age was reported at 37.0 weeks of gestation, and the weighted mean parity was observed at 4.0 [6].

Uterine atony was reported as the principal indication for PH, but it has changed toward abnormal placentation. Indications for PH are summarized in **Table 2** [6].

Differences in standards of antenatal care
Differences in standards of obstetric care
Differences in rates of cesarean delivery
Differences in parity, maternal age
Lack of blood banking facilities
Unavailability of advanced conservative interventional methods

Table 1.
Possible reasons for observed variations in incidences of PH.

Indication	%
Placental pathology	38
Abnormally invasive placenta	19
Placenta previa	10
Combined or unspecified placental pathology	8
Placental abruption or couvelaire uterus	1
Uterine atony	27
Uterine rupture	26
Unspecified hemorrhage	5
Infection	2
Cervical tear or laceration	1
Myomas or myomas with major obstetric hemorrhage	1
Disseminated intravascular coagulation	1
Hematoma	1
Abnormal pregnancy	1

Table 2.
Indications for PH.

An elective PH may be performed if abnormal placentation is diagnosed in the antepartum period. Occasionally pregnant women with stage IA2 and IB1 cervical carcinoma are candidates for an elective PH [11]. Severe postpartum infection unresponsive to medical therapy and placental site vessel subinvolution is other potential indications for elective PH [11–13]. Also, giving birth with cesarean section is associated with a fourfold risk compared to vaginal delivery [14].

4.1 Abnormal placentation

In addition, 59.8% of patients with adherent placenta and 75% with placenta previa have a history of previous cesarean section. The high incidence of PH is directly related to the increasing number of cesarean sections [15]. It has been reported that the incidence of placenta previa after one previous cesarean section increases by 47-fold in patients with four previous cesarean section [1]. Similarly, patients with previous surgical abortions were found to be more likely to have abnormal placentation. The risk is even higher in patients with multiple surgical abortions [16].

Multiparity
Oxytocin use for uterine stimulation
Preeclampsia
Multiple gestation
Prolonged labor

Table 3.
Independent risk factors for uterine atony.

Patients with only placenta previa have 16% risk of undergoing PH, but this risk rises up to 16% in patients with placenta previa and scarred uterus [17].

4.2 Uterine atony

While uterine atony was traditionally the most frequent indication for PH, its occurrence has declined due to newly developed pharmacological management facilities. Independent risk factors for uterine atony are listed in **Table 3** [14, 18].

4.3 Uterine rupture

11.4% to 45.5% of patients with uterine rupture may undergo PH. The risk factors for uterine rupture are multiple previous cesarean sections with a scarred uterus [1].

5. Preoperative evaluation

Even though it is a lifesaving operation, preoperative assessment techniques possess a key role in determining the success of the surgery. It is not always possible for the surgeon to take all the preventive measures before each case as the nature of the procedure is almost every time emergent. However, the factors listed below are recommended to be evaluated before each high-risk delivery:

1. Risk stratification: Preoperative planning and risk stratification models are essential to minimize the risk of undergoing hysterectomy and to reduce the morbidity associated with the procedure [19].

2. Clinical audit: Clinical audit can be used to evaluate the clinical management preceding peripartum hysterectomy and to determine if peripartum hysterectomies are potentially avoidable and by which means [20].

3. Imaging studies: In some cases, imaging studies such as ultrasound or MRI may be used to confirm the diagnosis or to identify the underlying cause of the bleeding [21].

4. Multidisciplinary approach: A multidisciplinary approach with ICU backup may improve outcomes [22].

5. Evaluation of risk factors: Evaluation of risk factors such as previous cesarean section, abnormal placentation, uterine atony, maternal coagulopathy, and maternal age may help in identifying women at high risk for peripartum hysterectomy.

6. Assessment of maternal and fetal risks and benefits: The decision to perform a peripartum hysterectomy should be made in consultation with a multidisciplinary team, including obstetricians, anesthesiologists, and hematologists, and should take into account the maternal and fetal risks and benefits [22].

6. Surgical technique

6.1 Position

Hysterectomy should be performed in the low lithotomy position. This position offers several advantages: (a) It allows for a thorough examination of patients with postpartum hemorrhage. It is an ideal position for identifying the source of bleeding. Lower genital tract lacerations and atonic bleeding are more easily recognized in this position. Additionally, transvaginal ultrasonography can be comfortably performed, facilitating the identification of upper intraperitoneal or extraperitoneal hematomas. (b) In cases of active bleeding, until the abdominal incision is initiated, this position enables the application of bimanual or vaginal tampons. (c) It is suitable for surgical interventions via the vaginal route. For cervical tears, cervical suturing can be performed, and in cases of deep vaginal tears, access to the pararectal or paravesical spaces can be achieved vaginally for necessary interventions and suturing. (d) This position provides advantages for surgical interventions via the abdominal route. Avascular spaces can be more easily accessed, allowing for better visualization of the topographic anatomy. This not only facilitates easier interventions but also reduces the risk of complications. Specifically, in cases with significant volume deficit requiring arterial ligation or placental invasion anomalies, this position is more advantageous for reducing bleeding and preventing complications. Furthermore, in placental invasion anomalies, the low lithotomy position is more beneficial during bladder dissection than the normal position.

6.2 Surgical site preparation

Povidone-iodine or chlorhexidine can be used for surgical site preparation. There is evidence suggesting the superiority of chlorhexidine, but these findings do not specifically pertain to postpartum hemorrhage surgery. It is known that the recovery of vaginal flora is parallel to vaginal cuff infections. Vaginal recolonization occurs more rapidly with chlorhexidine compared to povidone-iodine. Therefore, chlorhexidine can be used to reduce the risk of postoperative surgical site infections in these cases.

6.3 Antibiotic prophylaxis

The recommended regimen for prophylaxis is cefazolin 1 gram, and in cases where the surgical duration is prolonged, or the preoperative estimated blood loss exceeds 2 liters, or the intraoperative blood loss exceeds 2 liters, a 2-gram additional dose is advised.

6.4 Incision

The choice of incision is crucial for accessing the abdomen in the surgical management of postpartum hemorrhage. Especially in cases of placental invasion anomalies and complicated bleeding, a vertical incision is recommended to achieve complete and comfortable pelvic exposure. With this incision, dissection of the pelvic sidewall, particularly the vascular structures, can be performed more easily, and vascular clamping or ligations can be readily carried out. Additionally, preserving the integrity of the placenta is of utmost importance for the surgical management of placental invasion anomalies to prevent sudden bleeding. To achieve this, the fetus is delivered through an incision made from an area without the placenta, facilitated by the vertical incision. In cases of placenta accreta spectrum (PAS), after a vertical incision is made, the fetus is delivered through a fundal incision, ensuring the preservation of placental integrity and protecting the patient from sudden bleeding. In addition to these recommendations, experienced surgeons particularly prefer transverse incision in PAS cases. After entering the abdomen through a transverse incision, the fetus is delivered through a transverse incision just above the termination of the placenta. The remaining parts of the hysterectomy can be completed without compromising placental integrity. This technique can yield advantages such as reduced bleeding and improved cosmetic outcomes. Transverse incisions are also utilized in our clinic. For cases of uterine atony, a transverse incision is recommended. With this incision, procedures such as hysterectomy, arterial ligations, or compression sutures can be easily performed in cases of uterine atony. In situations where sufficient exposure is not achieved with the classic Pfannenstiel incision, relaxation of the rectus abdominis muscles can further facilitate access to the pelvis.

6.5 Retroperitoneal dissection with round ligament incision

During hysterectomy, the first structure usually incised is the round ligament. The round ligament incision allows for entry into the retroperitoneum by cutting the broad ligament parallel to the infundibulum of the ligament. Initially, the m. psoas muscle should be identified from this entry point. Then, the a. iliaca externa and v. iliaca externa, which run immediately medial to the muscle, should be easily located. Subsequently, the broad ligament is pushed medially, and separation from the external vascular structures is attempted. This enables the visualization of the ureter adhered to the broad ligament. Further dissection medially along the ureter reveals the a. iliaca interna just below, and entry into the pararectal avascular space between the a. iliaca interna and the ureter is achieved. This dissection allows for easy ligation of the a. iliaca interna for subsequent control of pelvic bleeding after hysterectomy. When following the a. iliaca interna anteriorly, the umbilical artery will be visible, and by dissecting the umbilical artery medially while keeping the a. and v. iliaca externa laterally, the paravesical space can be reached. In the inferior aspect of the paravesical space, the a. and v. obturatoria are found, while caudally, an aberrant v. obturatoria is present in approximately 30% of cases, along with the n. obturatorius in the inferior aspect. The exploration of this space also allows control over the paravaginal region in an inferio-caudal direction, facilitating the evacuation of hematomas, repair of tears, and suture ligation of ongoing bleeding in this area.

7. Special concerns

7.1 Total or subtotal hysterectomy?

Total abdominal hysterectomy is the procedure of choice, but subtotal PH may be a better choice in certain conditions where surgery needs to be completed in a shorter time. The advantages and disadvantages of subtotal PH are summarized in **Table 4** [1].

Advantages	Disadvantages
Lesser blood loss	Risk of malignancy in the residual stump
Reduced need for blood transfusion	Bleeding/discharge from residual stump
Reduced operating time	Need for regular cytology
Less intra and postoperative complications	Not effective in accreta in lower uterus

Table 4.
Advantages and disadvantages of subtotal PH.

Morbidity	%
Blood transfusion	88
Febrile episodes	26.5
Bladder injuries	8.8
DIC	
Ileus	
Vaginal cuff bleeding	
Adnexectomy	

Table 5.
Causes of morbidity with PH.

Both total and subtotal hysterectomy are associated with high morbidity and mortality [13]. Mean maternal mortality is reported to be about 4.8%. The causes of morbidity are listed in **Table 5** [17].

7.2 Role of vessel sealing devices

Based on the studies reviewed, vessel sealing devices have been shown to be effective and safe in achieving hemostasis during peripartum hysterectomies. They have been found to reduce operative time, blood loss, and the need for blood transfusions [23, 24]. Also, one of the studies claim they also reduce the number of intraoperative complications [23], while the other confines the benefit as not yet causing an increase [24]. The use of vessel sealing devices may be useful in both total and subtotal hysterectomies. However, it is important to note that vessel sealing devices should be used with caution and proper training to avoid complications such as thermal injury to adjacent tissues.

7.3 Who bleeds more?

Limited studies have been conducted to predict which cases are more prone to increased bleeding during peripartum hysterectomies. The data obtained from these studies are generally retrospectively designed due to ethical reasons and has limited evidence levels. However, it is known that the most effective factors contributing to increased bleeding are the necessity of performing hysterectomy in emergency conditions, limitations in preoperative preparations, and multidisciplinary approach.

As a notable finding, it has been observed that patients who have not previously undergone cesarean delivery surprisingly experience more bleeding during surgery.

Additionally, other factors that contribute to increased bleeding include the absence of intra-arterial balloon usage, the presence of known coagulation disorders in the patient, and awareness of the patient's desire to maintain fertility [25, 26].

For effective control of bleeding during peripartum hysterectomies, early diagnosis, appropriate interventions, and a multidisciplinary approach involving obstetricians, anesthesia specialists, and hematologists are important. However, further research and comprehensive studies are needed to better understand the risk factors for bleeding in peripartum hysterectomies and to develop management strategies.

7.4 Effect of body mass index

Class III obesity is an independent risk factor for increased morbidity at the time of peripartum hysterectomy, including the need for intensive care unit admission and readmission within 30 days [27]. According to the literature, although estimated blood loss and the number of transfusions do not differ depending on the patient's body mass index, there is a significant increase in surgical times and the number of wound infections.

7.5 Effect of assisted reproductive technologies

The role of assisted reproductive technologies (ART) in the risk of peripartum hysterectomies is a subject of study and debate. Although there is no consensus, several factors related to ART have been suggested as potential contributors to the increased risk of peripartum hysterectomies. Although the absolute risks are low, there is an almost fivefold increased risk of unplanned peripartum hysterectomy, and 1,7 more unplanned peripartum hysterectomies occur per 1000 deliveries in pregnancies with ART compared to those without ART. It is important to note that the exact contribution of ART to the risk of peripartum hysterectomies is still being researched, and individual cases may vary. Women undergoing ART should receive thorough prenatal care and should be closely monitored for potential complications [28, 29].

7.6 Preventive measures against venous thromboembolism (VTE)

Peripartum hysterectomy is associated with a significantly increased risk of VTE in the postpartum period, even when controlling for other known risk factors for postpartum thromboembolic events. The incidence of VTE following peripartum hysterectomy observed in a cross-sectional study with a big cohort shows that the population (2.2%) meets some guideline-based risk thresholds for routine thromboprophylaxis, potentially for at least two weeks postpartum. Further investigation into the role of routine VTE prophylaxis during and beyond the delivery encounter is needed [30].

7.7 Role of abdominal packing after peripartum hysterectomy

The scientific evidence suggests that abdominal packing can effectively control bleeding after peripartum hysterectomy in cases of intractable hemorrhage. Abdominal packing techniques include pads or roller gauze and balloon packs and abdominal packs retrieved within 24–48 hours. Studies have shown that abdominal packing can be successful in controlling bleeding after peripartum hysterectomy, even in cases where bleeding persists after the hysterectomy. However, there are potential risks associated with abdominal packing, such as infection and embolization of nontargeted vessels. The decision to use abdominal packing should be individualized based on the patient's clinical presentation and medical history [31, 32].

In a study that included more than a million deliveries consisting of 718 peripartum hysterectomies and 53 abdominal packing operations (about 1 per 14 hysterectomies), the success rate of abdominal packing was 62%, and the mortality rate was 24%. Other patients required other measures of interventions. The study concluded that abdominal packing was considerably helpful to physicians in means of being an option as a lifesaving procedure. The mean time for preserving the packing was 39 hours postpartum [31].

Some surgeons depend on modifications to abdominal packing procedures in the literature. In a six-patient case study, authors wrapped hot fluid-soaked and squeezed packing material circularly around a Bakri-type balloon and stabilized it, applying gentle pressure around the whole pelvic vasculature using the vaginal route. The estimated amount of bleeding was limited compared to the conventional packing procedure, and the method was useful in five patients [33].

7.8 Role of uterine compression sutures

The scientific evidence suggests that uterine compression sutures can effectively avoid cesarean hysterectomy in cases of intractable postpartum hemorrhage. Uterine compression sutures involve the placement of sutures around the uterus to compress the bleeding vessels and reduce bleeding. Several studies have evaluated the efficacy and safety of uterine compression sutures in preventing cesarean hysterectomy and reducing morbidity and mortality associated with postpartum hemorrhage. The benefits of uterine compression sutures include preservation of fertility, avoidance of hysterectomy, and ease of application. However, there are also potential risks associated with uterine compression sutures, such as infection, uterine rupture, and decidual cast formation [34].

Studies have shown that uterine compression sutures with additional hemostatic procedures can effectively control postpartum hemorrhage and prevent hysterectomy [35]. The B-Lynch suture technique and modified Pereira suture have also been reported to be effective alternatives to cesarean hysterectomy [36]. However, these methods are only recommended as first-line interruptions and will cause of losing valuable time during the management of patients with severe PAS and ones who already lost a considerable amount of blood.

7.9 Prophylactic intraoperative uterine artery embolization (UAE)

Prophylactic intraoperative uterine artery embolization during cesarean hysterectomy is a technique used to reduce the risk of intraoperative bleeding and complications in cases where cesarean delivery and subsequent hysterectomy are anticipated to be challenging or associated with a high risk of bleeding. The procedure involves the selective occlusion of the uterine arteries using embolic materials to decrease blood flow to the uterus.

The role of prophylactic intraoperative UAE is to limit blood loss during the surgical procedure by reducing blood flow to the uterus. By temporarily blocking the uterine arteries, the blood vessels that supply the uterus, the procedure aims to minimize the risk of excessive bleeding, which can be particularly challenging in cases of placenta accreta, increta, or percreta, where the placenta is abnormally attached to the uterine wall [37]. Several studies have evaluated the efficacy and safety of UAE in preventing cesarean hysterectomy and reducing morbidity and mortality associated with PAS [38]. The benefits of UAE include decreased blood loss, reduced morbidity, and preservation of fertility in some cases. However, there are also potential harms associated with UAE, such as the risk of embolization of nontargeted vessels, uterine necrosis, and infection [39].

7.10 Postoperative care

Based on the studies reviewed, the postoperative care measures after peripartum hysterectomy may include: (a) Monitoring for complications: Patients who undergo peripartum hysterectomy should be closely monitored for complications such as postoperative febrile illness, bladder injury, disseminated intravascular coagulation, acute kidney injury, wound infection, and maternal death. (b) Intensive care: A significant proportion of women who undergo peripartum hysterectomy may require intensive care postoperatively. (c) Correction of anemia: Correction of anemia before and after surgery may help to reduce the risk of complications and improve outcomes. (d) Blood transfusions: Liberal use of blood components may be necessary to manage hemorrhage and prevent complications. (e) Correction of coagulopathy: Correction of coagulopathy may be necessary to prevent bleeding and other complications. (f) Pain management: Adequate pain management should be provided to ensure patient comfort and facilitate recovery. (g) psychological support: Patients who undergo peripartum hysterectomy may experience anxiety and worry and may benefit from psychological support. (h) Follow-up care: Patients who undergo peripartum hysterectomy should receive appropriate follow-up care to monitor for complications and ensure optimal recovery. (i) Prevention of future complications: Measures to prevent future complications, such as improved antenatal care and identification of risk factors for peripartum hysterectomy, should be implemented [1, 9, 40].

7.11 Postoperative emotional burden

There is limited evidence on the emotional responses and depression after peripartum hysterectomy. However, some studies have reported on the postoperative complications and morbidity associated with peripartum hysterectomy, which may have an impact on emotional well-being [41, 42]. A study originated from a local nontertiary hospital reported on a surveillance questionnaire that indicated increased depression rates in peripartum hysterectomy patients compared to patients who had complicated cesarean deliveries [43]. Another questionnaire-based study showed women with peripartum hysterectomy had higher rates of emotional stress including fear, numbness, problems with bonding with the infant and delay in emotional reactions even after 6 months postpartum. All studies point out that women with peripartum hysterectomies need long-term psychological support [40].

Author details

Mehmet Baki Şentürk*, Çetin Çam and Batuhan Üstün
Namık Kemal University, Tekirdağ, Turkey

*Address all correspondence to: dr.baki77@gmail.com

References

[1] Machado LS. Emergency peripartum hysterectomy: Incidence, indications, risk factors and outcome. North American Journal of Medical Sciences. 2011;**3**(8):358-361

[2] Sharma B, Sikka P, Jain V, Jain K, Bagga R, Suri V. Peripartum hysterectomy in a tertiary care hospital: Epidemiology and outcomes. Journal of Anaesthesiology Clinical Pharmacology. 2017;**33**(3):324-328

[3] Smith J, Mousa HA. Peripartum hysterectomy for primary postpartum hemorrhage: Incidence and maternal morbidity. Journal of Obstetrics and Gynaecology. 2007;**27**(1):44-47

[4] Durfee RB. Evolution of cesarean hysterectomy. Clinical Obstetrics and Gynecology. 1969;**12**(3):575-589

[5] Chanrachakul B, Chaturachinda K, Phuapradit W, Roungsipragarn R. Cesarean and postpartum hysterectomy. International Journal of Gynaecology and Obstetrics. 1996;**54**(2):109-113

[6] van den Akker T, Brobbel C, Dekkers OM, Bloemenkamp KWM. Prevalence, indications, risk indicators, and outcomes of emergency Peripartum hysterectomy worldwide: A systematic review and meta-analysis. Obstetrics and Gynecology. 2016;**128**(6):1281-1294

[7] Whiteman MK, Kuklina E, Hillis SD, Jamieson DJ, Meikle SF, Posner SF, et al. Incidence and determinants of peripartum hysterectomy. Obstetrics and Gynecology. 2006;**108**(6):1486-1492

[8] Kwee A, Bots ML, Visser GH, Bruinse HW. Emergency peripartum hysterectomy: A prospective study in the Netherlands. European Journal of Obstetrics, Gynecology, and Reproductive Biology. 2006;**124**(2):187-192

[9] Athanasios FK, Alice M, Jakub D, Lotte Berdiin C, Catherine D-T, Serena D, et al. Epidemiological analysis of Peripartum hysterectomy across nine European countries. Acta Obstetricia Et Gynecologica Scandinavica. 2020;**99**(10):1364-1373

[10] Shravya G, Jason DW, Cande VA, Yongmei H, Mary ED, Alexander MF. Risk of Peripartum hysterectomy and Center hysterectomy and delivery volume. Obstetrics and Gynecology. 2016;**128**(6):1215-1224

[11] Ribeiro F, Correia L, Paula T, Santana I, Vieira Pinto L, Borrego J, et al. Cervical cancer in pregnancy: 3 cases, 3 different approaches. Journal of Lower Genital Tract Disease. 2013;**17**(1):66-70

[12] Anderson BL. Puerperal group a streptococcal infection: Beyond Semmelweis. Obstetrics and Gynecology. 2014;**123**(4):874-882

[13] Stokes M, Olson A, Algeo C, Rajab B, Mwalwanda C, Dongarwar D, et al. Clinical and sociodemographic characteristics associated with emergency Peripartum hysterectomy due to puerperal sepsis in Malawi. International Journal of Maternal and Child Health and AIDS. 2022;**11**(1):e535

[14] Sumaya H, Ian R, Bukola F, Rizwana C, Sabaratnam A, Haleema S. Risk factors for Peripartum hysterectomy among women with postpartum haemorrhage: Analysis of data from the WOMAN trial. BMC Pregnancy and Childbirth. 2018;**18**:186

[15] Yildirim GY, Koroglu N, Akca A, Talmac M, Dikmen S, Yildirim G, et al. What is new in peripartum hysterectomy? A seventeen year experience in a tertiary hospital. Taiwanese Journal of Obstetrics & Gynecology. 2021;**60**(1):95-98

[16] Ossola MW, Somigliana E, Mauro M, Acaia B, Benaglia L, Fedele L. Risk factors for emergency postpartum hysterectomy: The neglected role of previous surgically induced abortions. Acta Obstetricia et Gynecologica Scandinavica. 2011;**90**(12):1450-1453

[17] Christopoulos P, Hassiakos D, Tsitoura A, Panoulis K, Papadias K, Vitoratos N. Obstetric hysterectomy: A review of cases over 16 years. Journal of Obstetrics and Gynaecology. 2011;**31**(2):139-141

[18] Senturk MB, Cakmak Y, Guraslan H, Dogan K. Emergency peripartum hysterectomy: 2-year experiences in non-tertiary center. Archives of Gynecology and Obstetrics. 2015;**292**(5):1019-1025

[19] Sasirekha R, Saranya R, Sutharsika T. The changing scenario of pattern of Peripartum hysterectomy: Prevention and preparedness matters. International journal of reproduction contraception. Obstetrics and Gynecology. 2022;**11**(2):568-572

[20] Colmorn LB, Krebs L, Langhoff-Roos J, Group Ns. Potentially avoidable Peripartum hysterectomies in Denmark: A population based clinical audit. PLoS One. 2016;**11**(8):e0161302

[21] Seal SL, Kamilya G, Bhattacharyya SK, Mukherji J, Bhattacharyya AR. Relaparotomy after cesarean delivery: Experience from an Indian teaching hospital. The Journal of Obstetrics and Gynaecology Research. 2007;**33**(6):804-809

[22] Orsi M, Ossola MW, Iurlaro E, Perugino G, Somigliana E, Ferrazzi E. The impact of a multilevel approach to reduce emergency hysterectomy for postpartum haemorrhage: Insights from a tertiary referral Centre in northern Italy. European Journal of Obstetrics, Gynecology, and Reproductive Biology. 2022;**271**:152-157

[23] Lauroy A, Verhaeghe C, Vidal F, Parant O, Legendre G, Guerby P. Perioperative outcomes using LigaSure compared with conventional technique in peripartum hysterectomy. Archives of Gynecology and Obstetrics. 2020;**301**(1):229-234

[24] Rossetti D, Vitale SG, Bogani G, Rapisarda AM, Gulino FA, Frigerio L. Usefulness of vessel-sealing devices for peripartum hysterectomy: A retrospective cohort study. Updates in Surgery. 2015;**67**(3):301-304

[25] Takahashi H, Ohkuchi A, Usui R, Suzuki H, Baba Y, Matsubara S. Factors contributing to massive blood loss on Peripartum hysterectomy for abnormally invasive placenta: Who bleeds more? Obstetrics and Gynecology International. 2016;**2016**:5349063

[26] de la Cruz CZ, Thompson EL, O'Rourke K, Nembhard WN. Cesarean section and the risk of emergency peripartum hysterectomy in high-income countries: A systematic review. Archives of Gynecology and Obstetrics. 2015;**292**(6):1201-1215

[27] Wortman AC, Hernandez JS, Holcomb DS, Wilson KL, McIntire DD, Sheffield JS. Effect of body mass index on maternal morbidity following peripartum hysterectomy. Clinical Obesity. 2015;**5**(2):72-78

[28] Park HS, Kwon H, McElrath TF. Assisted reproductive technology and

the risk of unplanned peripartum hysterectomy: Analysis using propensity score matching. Human Reproduction. 2018;**33**(8):1466-1473

[29] Cromi A, Candeloro I, Marconi N, Casarin J, Serati M, Agosti M, et al. Risk of peripartum hysterectomy in births after assisted reproductive technology. Fertility and Sterility. 2016;**106**(3):623-628

[30] Mauney L, Barth WH Jr, Clapp MA. Association between peripartum hysterectomy and venous thromboembolism. American Journal of Obstetrics and Gynecology. 2022;**226**(1):119 e1-119e11

[31] Deffieux X, Vinchant M, Wigniolle I, Goffinet F, Sentilhes L. Maternal outcome after abdominal packing for uncontrolled postpartum hemorrhage despite peripartum hysterectomy. PLoS One. 2017;**12**(6):e0177092

[32] Yoong W, Lavina A, Ali A, Sivashanmugarajan V, Govind A, McMonagle M. Abdomino-pelvic packing revisited: An often forgotten technique for managing intractable venous obstetric haemorrhage. The Australian & New Zealand Journal of Obstetrics & Gynaecology. 2019;**59**(2):201-207

[33] Kilicci C, Polat M, Kucukbas M, Senturk MB, Karakus R, Yayla Abide C, et al. Modified abdominal packing method in "near miss" patients with postpartum hemorrhages. Turkish Journal Of Obstetrics And Gynecology. 2018;**15**(3):159-164

[34] Moleiro ML, Braga J, Machado MJ, Guedes-Martins L. Uterine compression sutures in controlling postpartum haemorrhage: A narrative review. Acta Médica Portuguesa. 2022;**35**(1):51-58

[35] Kwong LT, So PL, Wong SF. Uterine compression sutures with additional hemostatic procedures for the management of postpartum hemorrhage. The Journal of Obstetrics and Gynaecology Research. 2020;**46**(11):2332-2339

[36] Moleiro ML, Guedes-Martins L, Mendes A, Marques C, Braga J. Modified Pereira suture as an effective option to treat postpartum Hemorrhage due to uterine atony. Revista Brasileira de Ginecologia e Obstetrícia. 2018;**40**(2):92-95

[37] Li Q, Yang ZQ, Mohammed W, Feng YL, Shi HB, Zhou X. Prophylactic uterine artery embolization assisted cesarean section for the prevention of intrapartum hemorrhage in high-risk patients. Cardiovascular and Interventional Radiology. 2014;**37**(6):1458-1463

[38] Yuan Q, Jin Y, Chen L, Ling L, Bai XM. Prophylactic uterine artery embolization during cesarean delivery for placenta previa complicated by placenta accreta. International Journal of Gynaecology and Obstetrics. 2020;**149**(1):43-47

[39] Sivan E, Spira M, Achiron R, Rimon U, Golan G, Mazaki-Tovi S, et al. Prophylactic pelvic artery catheterization and embolization in women with placenta accreta: Can it prevent cesarean hysterectomy? American Journal of Perinatology. 2010;**27**(6):455-461

[40] de la Cruz CZ, Coulter ML, O'Rourke K, Amina Alio P, Daley EM, Mahan CS. Women's experiences, emotional responses, and perceptions of care after emergency peripartum hysterectomy: A qualitative survey of women from 6 months to 3 years postpartum. Birth. 2013;**40**(4):256-263

[41] Zaat TR, van Steijn ME, de Haan-Jebbink JM, Olff M, Stramrood CAI, van Pampus MG. Posttraumatic stress disorder related to postpartum haemorrhage: A systematic review. European Journal of Obstetrics, Gynecology, and Reproductive Biology. 2018;**225**:214-220

[42] van Steijn ME, Scheepstra KWF, Zaat TR, van der Post JAM, Olff M, van Pampus MG. Posttraumatic stress disorder in partners following severe postpartum haemorrhage: A prospective cohort study. Women and Birth. 2020;**33**(4):360-366

[43] Senturk MB, Cakmak Y, Ozalp A. Postpartum depression and associated factors after emergency peripartum hysterectomy. The Journal of the Pakistan Medical Association. 2017;**67**(1):49-53

Chapter 3

3D Total Laparoscopic Hysterectomy of a Very Large Uterine Myoma in a Super Morbidly Obese Woman of Body Mass Index 60 Kg/m^2: A Case Report and a Literature Review

Sharifah Halimah Jaafar, Iskandar Khalid and Shahridan Mohd Fathil

Abstract

A 40-year-old Malay nulliparous female, morbidly obese (height 161 cm, weight 158.5 kg, BMI 60.1 kg/m^2) presented with a large uterine fibroid, FIGO Grade 4 with its upper border extending up to the 4 cm above the umbilicus. After 6 months of GnRH suppression, she consented to a total laparoscopic hysterectomy. Preoperatively, she was optimized, and bowel preparation was done with 3 days of liquid diet, a rectal enema, and antacid pre-induction. A nasogastric tube was inserted before port entry. The ports were placed higher, with the primary port at the epigastric region and the working ports on the left paramedian at the level of the umbilicus and ipsilateral left lumbar. Intracorporeal myomectomy was done to reduce the mass size before proceeding to a total hysterectomy in the usual manner. The patient was stable throughout the operation, and blood loss was approximately 900 mls. Postoperatively, the patient was fully ambulated and resumed a regular diet 24 hours after surgery, and was discharged home well. Operating a sizeable uterine mass in a super-morbidly obese woman laparoscopically is technically far more challenging for surgical and anesthetic management. Perioperative preparation, positioning, anesthetic management, and ergonomic port placement are paramount to surgical outcomes. Minimally invasive surgery is safe and feasible, and it is the best option for the morbidly obese patients as it allows early mobilization and spares them from tumultuous postoperative morbidity from open surgery, as proven by our case.

Keywords: super-morbid obesity, large uterine fibroid, total hysterectomy, 3D total laparoscopic hysterectomy, minimally invasive surgery

1. Introduction

In the past, laparoscopic surgery was considered a relative contraindication in obese patients. However, since the feasibility of performing laparoscopy on the obese patient was first published in the gynecologic literature in 1976 [1–3], there have been increasing evidence that obese patients benefit from laparoscopic surgery compared to the abdominal approach [4, 5]. However, data on patients with a BMI of 40 are limited.

On the other hand, laparoscopic hysterectomy of a huge uterine mass is technically challenging, but it has been proven feasible and safe procedure if performed by experienced surgeons regardless of the size, number, and location without much morbidity [6–9].

However, operating a large uterine mass in a super-morbidly obese woman laparoscopically is technically far more challenging for surgical and anesthetic management. Still, it is the best option for the patient as it allows early mobilization and spares them from tumultuous postoperative morbidity from open surgery. We are reporting a case of total laparoscopic hysterectomy for a large uterine mass of 24 weeks gestation in a super morbidly obese woman with a body mass index of 60 kg/m^2. To our knowledge, this combination of sizeable uterine mass in a super-morbidly obese woman successfully managed laparoscopically is rarely reported.

2. Case presentation

A 40-year-old Malay nulliparous female (Height 161 cm, Weight 158.5 kg, BMI 60.1 kg/m^2) presented with a history of severe menorrhagia for 6 months. She had been on medical treatment, an injection of Leuprolide acetate and progestin to control the bleeding symptoms; however, she opted for earlier surgical intervention due to intolerable side effects. She was morbidly obese with massive central adiposity on the chest, abdomen, and thigh. She also has bilateral lower limbs and chronic venous insufficiency evident by the varicose veins and leathery hyperpigmented skin of her lower extremities from mid-shin to the ankles bilaterally (**Figure 1**).

The patient's past medical and surgical history was unremarkable. Physical examination revealed a pelvic-abdominal mass with the upper border extending up

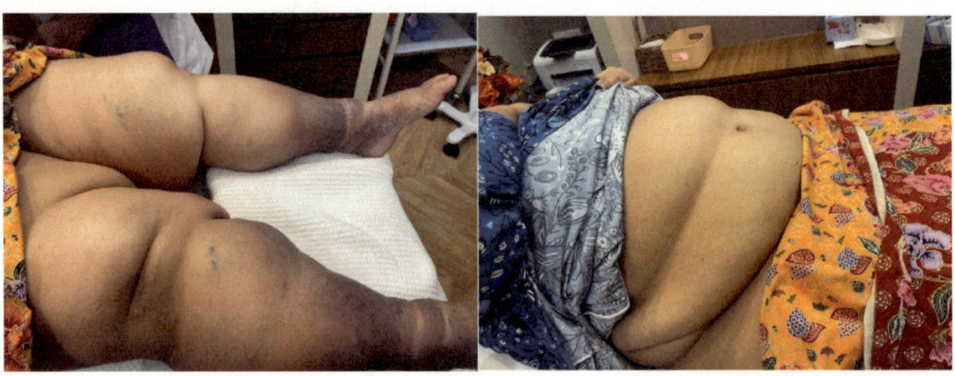

Figure 1.
The patient's thick abdominal wall with bilateral lower limbs chronic venous insufficiency is evident by the varicose veins and leathery hyperpigmented skin of her lower extremities from mid-shin to the ankles.

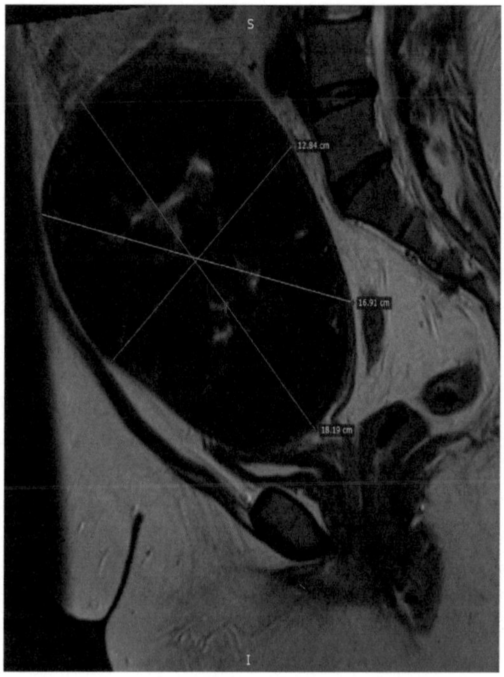

Figure 2.
The magnetic resonance imaging (MRI) examination showed features of left lower anterior lateral large uterine leiomyoma measuring 182 × 128 × 169 mm (ap x w x cc), FIGO grade 4-5 compressing the bladder inferiorly.

to 4 cm above the umbilicus. An ultrasound was performed both abdominally and vaginally. It showed a vast uterine with a large single oval-shaped encapsulated mass likely to be a uterine fibroid, FIGO Grade 4, arising from the lower segment of the anterior-lateral aspect of the uterus, pushing the uterine fundus up, and deviating to the right. The magnetic resonance imaging (MRI) examination showed features of left lower anterior lateral large uterine leiomyoma measuring 182 × 128 × 169 mm (ap x w x cc), FIGO Grade 4-5 compressing the bladder inferiorly (**Figure 2**). There were no features suggestive of malignancy. Her pap smear and endometrial sampling results were both routine. Her preoperative hemoglobin was 11.9 g%. An option of bariatric surgery to manage her weight was discussed; however, she opted for a total laparoscopic hysterectomy.

The patient was counseled about the risks of morcellation of potential occult uterine leiomyosarcoma (LMS) or smooth muscle tumors of uncertain malignant potential. Written informed consent was obtained for the procedure and the publication of the case report and the accompanying images.

3. Perioperative preparation and management

She was asked to take only a liquid diet 3 days before admission for surgery. Preoperatively, bowel preparation was performed by giving a rectal enema the night before surgery. A bolus of intravenous Esomeprazole 40 mg was given before induction as a prophylaxis to gastric acid aspiration in anticipation of difficult intubation.

The patient was assessed preoperatively 1 week before the surgery. Upon arrival to the operating room, the patient was placed in the head elevated laryngoscopy position using the Troop Elevation Pillow for induction. A 20G peripheral venous access was initially obtained at her left antecubital fossa under ultrasound guidance and another 18G cannula at her right-hand post-induction (**Figure 3**).

The patient was ventilated using pressure-regulated volume control with a tidal volume of 320 ml, that is 6 ml/kg ideal body weight, generating peak airway pressure of 35 mm Hg, adequate to maintain ventilation with an end-tidal carbon dioxide value of 45 to 55 mmHg throughout pneumoperitoneum and surgery.

TCI propofol and remifentanil maintenance was at 3 µcg/ml and 8 ng/ml on average for maintenance titrated to an anesthetic depth bispectral Index (BIS) value of 40 to 60. A profound neuromuscular blockade was maintained throughout surgery and titrated to a neuromuscular monitoring (NMT) Tain-of-Four (TOF) ratio of 0/4. Multimodal analgesia with intravenous paracetamol, intravenous oxycodone 10 mg toward the end of the surgery, intravenous parecoxib 40 mg immediately after the surgery, and intravenous palanosetron 0.75 mg, and dexamethasone 8 mg were administered for postoperative nausea and vomiting prophylaxis.

Other than a brief period of hypotension post-induction, blood pressure and pulse rate were within 20% of the patient's baseline throughout the operation. She was given 3 liters of sterofundin and 1 liter of gelafusine with an estimated blood loss of 1 liter. Adequate urine output of 0.5 ml/kg/hr. was maintained throughout the surgery.

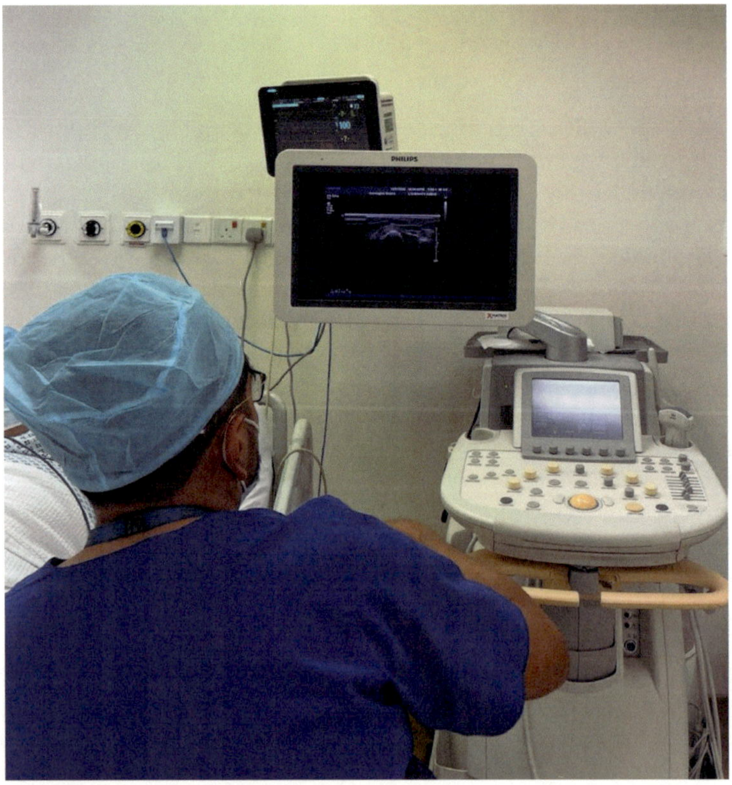

Figure 3.
The anesthetist establishes peripheral venous access at her left antecubital fossa under ultrasound guidance to locate the vein.

4. Surgery and positioning

Following induction of anesthesia, the patient's arms were tucked to her sides. She was secured in a low lithotomy position with liberal padding on the legs and arms (**Figure 4**). Additionally, stationary shoulder blocks were placed to maintain her at a 20-degree tilt in the Trendelenburg position. The bladder was emptied, and a naso-gastric tube was inserted to ensure the stomach was not distended during trocar entry. We failed to place a uterine manipulator (RUMI®II Koh-Efficient system) into the uterine cavity due to obstruction of the endocervical canal and extreme deviation of the cervix to the right by the large mass.

Abdominal entry & port placement: Pneumoperitoneum is established using ENDOPATH® insufflation Needle Ultra Veress (UV120, 120 mm) inserted *via* intra-umbilicus (the thinnest skin-peritoneum distance), with insufflation pressure of 20 mmHg. The primary port was positioned on the midline of Le Hwang, slightly below the epigastrium, by using an Endopath Xcel® dilating tip trocar (100 × 12 mm, Ethicon® Endo-Surgery), which was driven into an incision against the abdominal pressure. The intraabdominal pressure was reduced to 16 mmHg and maintained throughout the surgery. Intra-abdominal visualization was achieved using a 12 mm, 30° telescope (Karl Storz, 4 K RUBINA ® 3D Telescope system). Three 5 mm ancillary ports were positioned on the left iliac fossa, the left paramedian at the level of the umbilicus lateral to the border of the rectus abdominis muscle, and the right

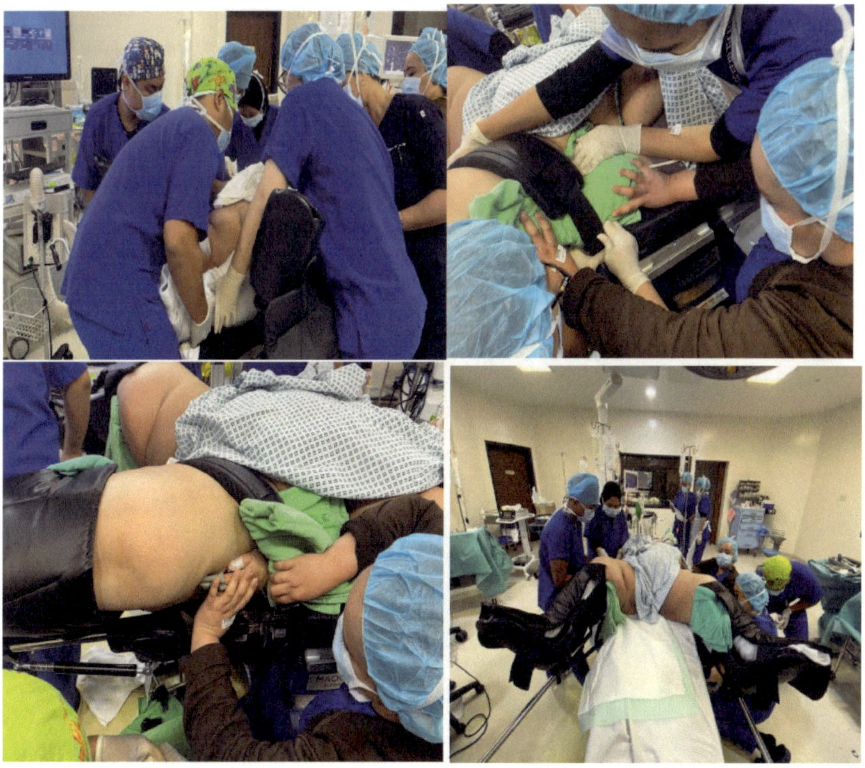

Figure 4.
Following the induction of anesthesia, the patient's arms were tucked to her sides. She was secured in a low lithotomy position with liberal padding on the legs and arms to prevent pressure necrosis and tractional nerve injury.

iliac fossa in parallel with the left side using Endopath Xcel® dilating tip trocar (100 × 5 mm, Ethicon Endo-Surgery) inserted under direct visualization of the telescope (**Figure 5**). The surgical table was tilted and placed a 15–20° head-down Trendelenburg position as agreeable by the anesthesiologist.

The operation: We used Maryland LigaSure™ Smart Bipolar forceps (36 cm × 5 mm) in this procedure for coagulation and cutting the pedicles and fibers throughout the procedure, bipolar Robby Kelly grasping forceps (Karl-Storz, 3.5 × 200 mm) to seal the vessels, and monopolar powered hook (Kar-Storz, 3.5 × 200 mm) for dissection. The first stage of the surgery involved freeing the large mass from the adhesion to the sigmoid colon (**Figure 6**) and freeing the sigmoid colon from its natural fixation to allow its mobilization to the upper abdomen.

We started with coagulating and transecting the ovarian pedicles and the round ligaments bilaterally with Maryland LigaSure™ forceps to improve the mobility of the uterus and reduce the blood flow. Attempt to approach and seal the uterine artery from its origin from medial and lateral approaches failed due to the obstructing large uterine mass limiting the space for maneuvering to the lateral spaces. At this juncture, due to a sizeable anterior fibroid obstructing the view to the pelvis and pelvic side wall, we decided to perform a myomectomy to reduce the size of the mass to facilitate handling and permit a view of the pelvis and lower part of the uterus (**Figure 7**). To control the blood loss, 40 ml of vasopressin (20 units in 100 ml saline) was injected into the fibroid capsule. A sizeable transverse incision was made across the anterior surface of the uterus. With the help of a myoma screw and the grasping forceps to countertraction, the monopolar powered hook and scissor were used to cut the fibers. The large myoma was finally enucleated with some difficulty due to its large size, location involving the

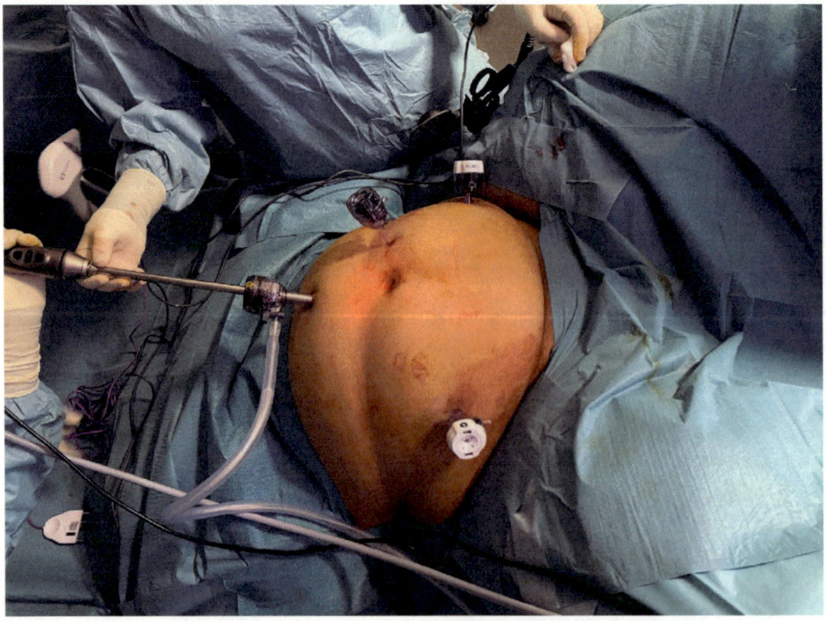

Figure 5.
The primary port was positioned on the midline of Le Hwang, slightly below the epigastrium, by using an Endopath Xcel® dilating tip trocar (100 × 12 mm, Ethicon® Endo-surgery). Three 5 mm ancillary ports were positioned on the left iliac fossa, the left paramedian at the level of the umbilicus lateral to the border of the rectus abdominis muscle, and the right iliac fossa in parallel with the left side using Endopath Xcel® dilating tip trocar (100 × 5 mm, Ethicon Endo-Surgery) inserted under direct visualization of the telescope.

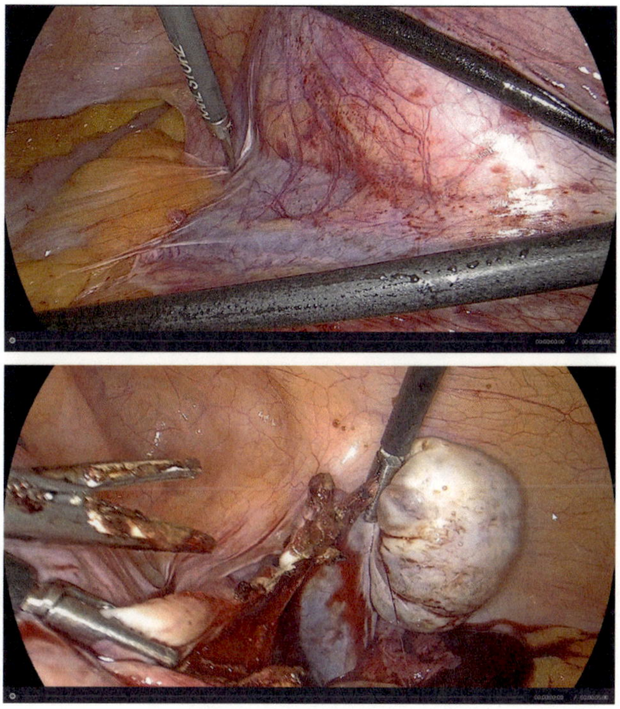

Figure 6.
(a) Shows the first stage of the surgery involved freeing the large mass from the adhesion to the sigmoid colon. (b) Shows the transaction of the ovarian ligament from the uterus.

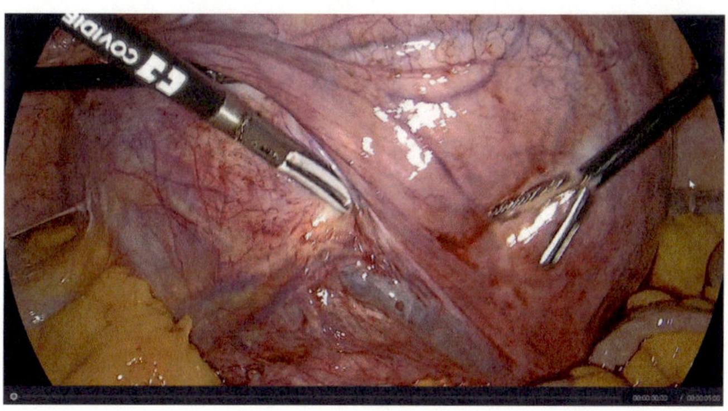

Figure 7.
A sizeable anterior fibroid obstructing the view to the pelvis and pelvic side wall.

anterior lower segment of the uterus, and its fibrotic surgical plane **Figure 8**). The bleeders and hemostasis were handled and secured with suturing and bipolar coagulation.

Following the myomectomy, the uterine manipulator (RUMI®II Koh-Efficient system) was successfully placed into the uterine cavity to manipulate the smaller uterus. We continued the dissection anteriorly from the round ligaments down to the vesicouterine peritoneal fold to find the correct plane. The course of the ureters was identified. With the help of a uterine manipulator, which pushes the uterus cephalad and away from the ureters, the ascending branch of the uterine vessels was ligated with a suture and divided at the level of the isthmus of the uterus (**Figure 9**).

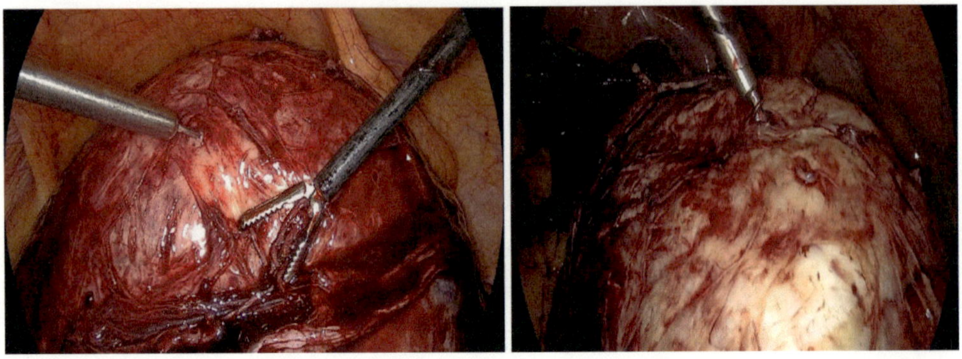

Figure 8.
(a) Shows the injection of vasopressin (20 units in 100 ml saline) into the fibroid capsule to reduce blood loss. (b) With the help of a myoma screw, the grasping forceps to countertraction, and the monopolar powered hook to cut the fibers, the large myoma was enucleated with some difficulty due to its large size, location involving the lower segment, and its fibrotic surgical plane.

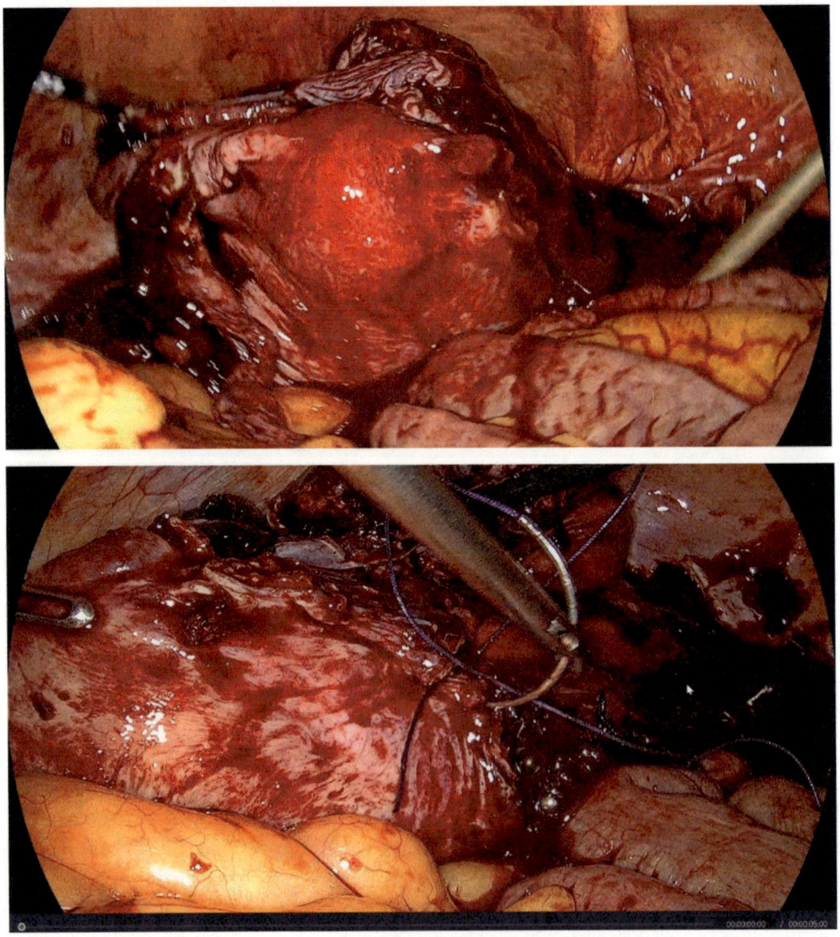

Figure 9.
(a) Shows the image of the uterus after myomectomy. (b) With the help of a uterine manipulator, which pushes the uterus cephalad and away from the ureters, the ascending branch of the uterine vessels was ligated with a suture and divided at the level of the isthmus of the uterus.

The bladder flab was pushed downward, and the anterior cervical fascia was exposed for dissection of the cervix below the cervicovaginal margin. The cardinal ligament fibers were incised posteriorly to the uterosacral ligaments and inferiorly, identifying the lowest limit of dissection as the cervicovaginal margin. The colpotomy was completed by incising the vagina with a monopolar-powered hook at the precise margin of the cervix along the impression of the rim of the RUMI's cup in the vagina. The smaller uterus was retrieved from the abdominal cavity through the vagina. However, due to a narrowed vagina, the large myoma was morcellated with Versator ™powered morcellator uncontained. In this case, it was challenging to do in-bag morcellation of the fibroid due to its large size, limited space of the abdominal cavity, and thick abdominal wall. The morcellated myoma was extracted *via* the left iliac fossa port under direct visualization of the telescope (**Figure 10**). The vaginal cuff was laparoscopically sutured with the Vicryl 1/0 suture continuously. There were no complications; the operating time was approximately 485 min. Intraoperative blood loss was about 900 ml. The final weight of the removed morcellated uterus with myoma was 1210 g (300 × 300 × 120 cm), and the findings of the pathologic examination were consistent with a benign fibroid uterus.

5. Postoperative care

The postanaesthetic care unit (PACU) stay was uneventful with stable hemodynamic parameters, pulse oximetry of 100%, and a pain score of 1/10. Venous thromboembolic prophylaxis in stockings and subcutaneous low-molecular-weight heparin was utilized, and incentive spirometry was initiated on the first postoperative day. The patient's diet slowly advanced within 12 hours after surgery, and she was discharged from the hospital within 24 hours of the procedure in a satisfactory condition (**Figure 11**).

6. Discussion

Traditionally, laparoscopic surgery was not recommended for individuals with obesity; nevertheless, recent research indicates that employing a minimally invasive approach for gynecological procedures in obese and severely obese patients (those with a body mass index, or BMI, of ≥35 kg/m^2) yields superior outcomes compared to the conventional abdominal approach [3]. This approach has been proven feasible and is associated with reduced rates of postoperative complications such as shorter recovery periods, decreased hospital stays, diminished postoperative discomfort, lower instances of surgical site infections, venous thromboembolism, wound complications, reduced risk of hernias, and improved cosmetic results [7].

While preoperative weight reduction is the ideal course of action for severely obese patients needing gynecological surgery, it is often challenging to achieve. Performing laparoscopic surgery on a substantial uterine mass can pose technical challenges, particularly when surgical access is restricted due to excess intra-abdominal fat and the size of the uterine mass. However, with a well-considered surgical strategy encompassing preoperative planning and postoperative care, it can be successfully accomplished.

In this case, a super-morbidly obese woman with a body mass index, BMI 60 kg/m^2 with a large uterine mass underwent a total laparoscopic hysterectomy (TLH), although

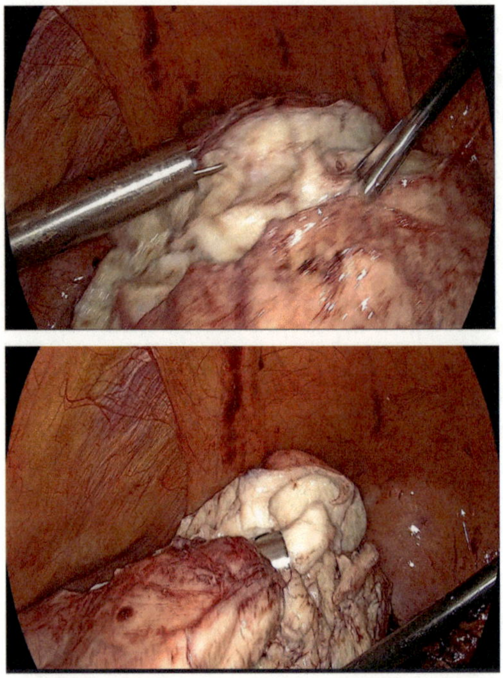

(a)

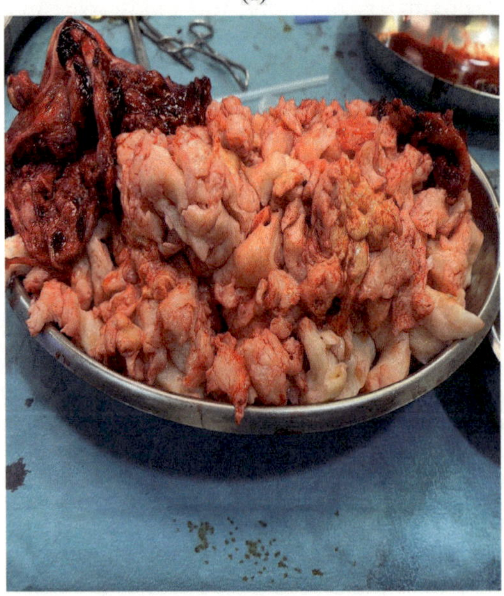

(b)

Figure 10.
(a) Shows the uncontained large myoma was morcellated with Versator ™powered morcellator. The morcellated myoma was extracted via the left iliac fossa port under direct visualization of the telescope. In this case, it was challenging to do in-bag morcellation of the fibroid due to its large size to fit the bag, limited space of the abdominal cavity, and thick abdominal wall. (b) Shows the morcellated myoma and the uterus extracted from the abdomen. The final weight of the removed morcellated uterus with myoma was 1210 g (300 × 300 × 120 cm).

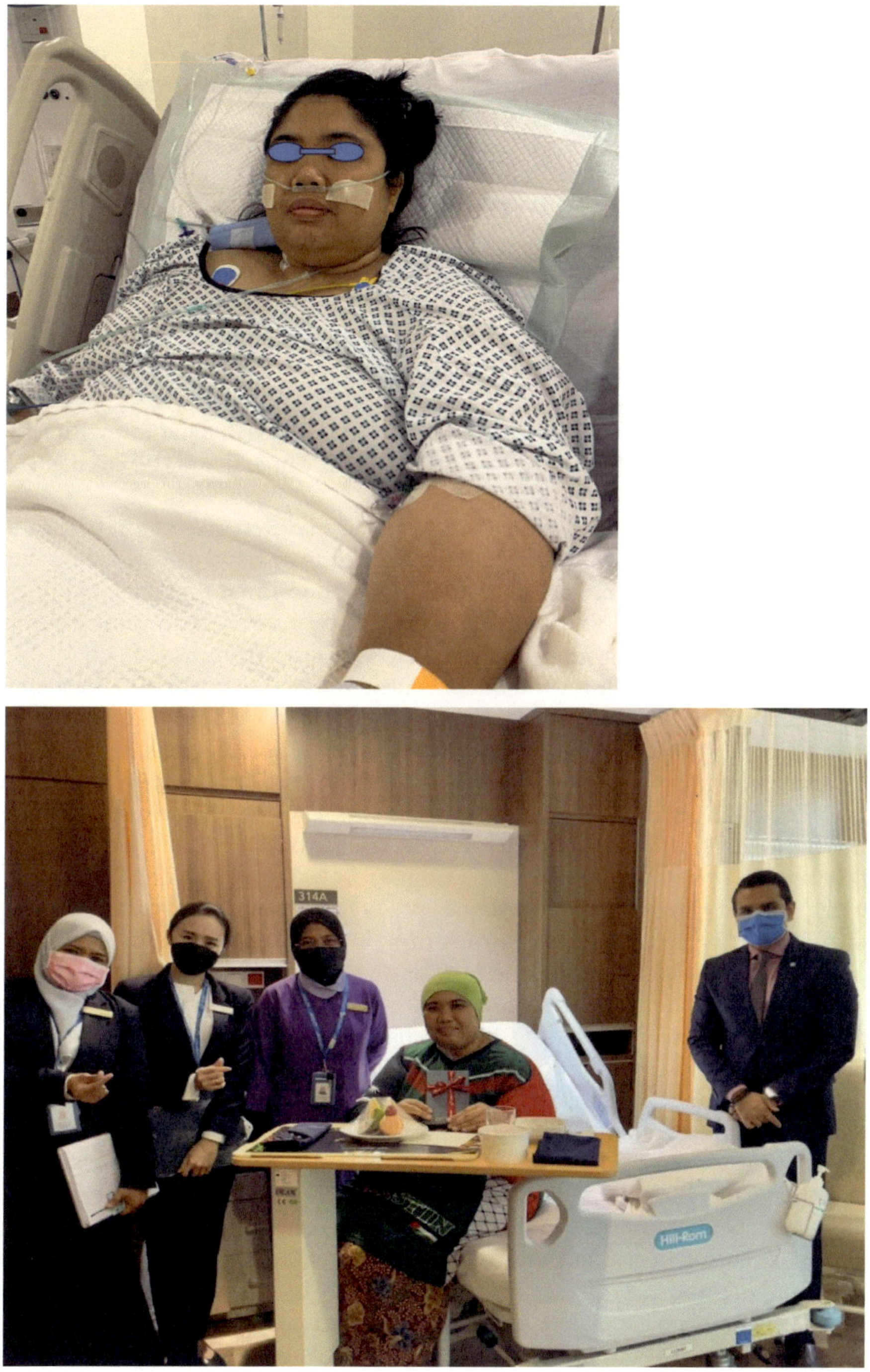

Figure 11.
(a) Shows the patient is comfortable at 6 hours after surgery in high-dependency unit. (b) The patient's diet slowly advanced within 12 hours after surgery, and she was discharged from the hospital within 24 hours of the procedure in satisfactory condition. (Photos shown with permission from the patient).

it took longer operative times; the operation was successful with no complications and postoperative morbidity. This case highlights the feasibility of laparoscopic surgery, and the technical challenges that surgeons may encounter when operating on a large uterine mass in an extremely obese patient.

Preoperative optimization is critical to ensure a safe surgical outcome in the morbidly obese. Preoperatively, obese patients should be thoroughly evaluated utilizing the New York Heart Association (NYHA) classification and the American Society of Anesthesiologists (ASA) score for any comorbidities affecting anesthetic management such as obstructive sleep apnea, diabetes, hypertension, and cardiovascular diseases [10, 11].

Preoperative mechanical bowel preparation for TLH has not been shown in randomized control studies to be beneficial in improving intraoperative visualization, bowel handling, or overall ease of performing the procedure [12]. However, in a complex case, in particular, operating a large uterine mass in a patient with excess visceral fat, as in our case, it might be helpful when the bowel and the stomach are decompressed to prevent inadvertent injury.

Proper patient positioning during induction and maintenance of anesthesia is also paramount important as obese patients are more prone to airway obstruction due to increased upper airway collapsibility and higher abdominal pressure [13]. Video laryngoscopy and awake intubation techniques may be necessary in some cases to improve airway visualization and reduce the risk of complications [14, 15].

Intraoperatively, maintaining adequate ventilation and oxygenation is crucial to prevent anesthesia-related complications, such as hypoxemia and respiratory acidosis [16]. Strategies to optimize lung function, such as positive end-expiratory pressure (PEEP) and recruitment maneuvers, may be necessary to improve oxygenation and reduce postoperative pulmonary complications [13]. Close monitoring of hemodynamic parameters, fluid management, and electrolyte balance is also essential in obese patients to prevent cardiovascular and metabolic complications [14].

During a total laparoscopic hysterectomy (TLH), patients are typically placed in the dorsal lithotomy or Trendelenburg position, inclined at an angle of 15–20 degrees. This positioning risks patient displacement or potential neurologic injuries [17]. To secure patients effectively in the Trendelenburg position, it is essential to provide leg support, ample arm and leg padding, stable shoulder blocks, and bean bags [16].

Additionally, although uncommon, nerve injuries to the upper and lower extremities are potential complications of laparoscopic gynecological surgery [17, 16]. To minimize the risk of unintended brachial plexus injuries, it is advisable to either tuck the patient's arms at their sides or limit arm abduction to less than 90 degrees when using extended arm boards [17].

The lithotomy position has also been associated with nerve injuries in the lower extremities, affecting nerves such as the femoral, lateral femoral cutaneous, sciatic, obturator, and common peroneal nerves, particularly in surgeries lasting longer than 2 hours [17]. Therefore, especially in super-obese patients, it is crucial to reduce the risk of neurologic injuries in the lower extremities through meticulous positioning and the use of booted stirrups to alleviate external pressure on the legs during the surgical procedure.

Abdominal entry and establishing a pneumoperitoneum can pose significant challenges when dealing with super-obese patients with large uterine masses. To enhance the success rate while minimizing complications, a strategy involves realigning the umbilical axis and initiating insufflation at a higher pressure, typically ranging from 20 to 25 mmHg, with a rapid flow rate. This approach has shown promise in reducing complications such as preperitoneal insufflation, subcutaneous emphysema, visceral injury, vascular injury, penetration of an underlying skin fold, and postoperative wound complications [18].

In our specific case, where the uterine mass extended beyond the umbilicus, we successfully employed the Le Hwang line—a midline point between the umbilicus and the epigastrium—for abdominal entry. This was achieved using a 12 mm bladed trocar under an insufflation pressure of 20 mmHg. Using an optical access trocar can further enhance safety during abdominal entry, significantly lowering the risk of iatrogenic injuries [19].

Furthermore, in morbidly obese patients, access to deep pelvic structures and optimal visceral exposure can be compromised due to the increased thickness of the abdominal wall and excess intraabdominal adiposity [20, 21]. In cases involving large uterine masses, placing the working port higher along a diagonal line with the primary port, on the same side as the surgeon, has proven to provide better ergonomics for instrument handling and maneuvering toward the target area. Considering that standard laparoscopic instruments typically measure 33 cm, using bariatric instruments, which can extend up to 45 cm in length, offers improved access to deeper pelvic structures in morbidly obese patients, particularly when performing colpotomy procedures.

Performing a laparoscopic hysterectomy for a benign, large uterine mass can present technical challenges, particularly when it resides in the lower segment or extends into the broad ligament. Such masses tend to occupy the pelvis, making it difficult to visualize vital anatomical structures like the ureters. This can pose a risk of difficulty in accessing anatomical planes, potentially leading to hemorrhage or organ injury. Nevertheless, with the right strategy and technique, laparoscopic hysterectomy remains a safe and feasible option [6, 10].

In our case, we employed a technique described in the literature [6, 22], which involved intraoperative myomectomy to decompress the large uterus (as illustrated in **Figure 8a** and **b**) before proceeding with the hysterectomy. This approach is particularly useful when dealing with a large myoma located anteriorly, obstructing the vesicouterine reflection, complicating bladder dissection, or in cases with a sizable broad ligament fibroid, where normalization of anatomy is necessary before hysterectomy. In our specific case, given the substantial size and weight of the fibroid, we utilized a myoma screw through one of the 5 mm ancillary ports to apply traction and countertraction forces, facilitating the separation of the myoma from the uterus. Once the large myoma is successfully separated, the hysterectomy can proceed as usual.

Extracting a large specimen through the thick abdominal wall and a constricted vaginal canal can pose technical challenges. In our case, the smaller uterus was morcellated using a size 9 scalpel blade through the vagina, while the large myoma specimen was morcellated using a power morcellator (uncontained) through the left lumbar port site. It is worth noting that there is increasing evidence suggesting that intra-abdominal specimen morcellation is associated with a heightened risk of spreading occult cancerous tissues beyond the abdominal cavity, potentially impacting patient prognosis [23].

Similarly, when using the transvaginal approach for uterus specimen extraction, it may necessitate segmental resection, split-half resection, or piecemeal resection of the uterus, depending on its size and shape, due to the limited operative field. Consequently, the partially cut surface of the uterine body may be exposed to the pelvic cavity, and fragmental tissue resulting from piecemeal resection of the large uterine body might also enter the pelvic cavity. Therefore, if uterine sarcomas are present, involvement of the abdominal and pelvic cavities may be unavoidable following the transvaginal removal of a large uterus [24]. Hence, comprehensive preoperative evaluation is crucial to minimize or exclude the possibility of potential malignant tumors, and obtaining informed consent from the patient is paramount.

In conclusion, there is an anticipated increase in the number of severely obese patients undergoing TLH. This trend will present specific physiological and technical difficulties that surgeons should be ready to address. However, TLH remains a secure, feasible, and practical approach to gynecologic surgery for morbidly obese patients with reasonable uterine size and has demonstrated low complication rates. A thorough preoperative risk assessment, optimizing patient's condition, implementing careful strategy of, TLH procedure, plus a meticulous postoperative care, are paramount importance as minimal-access surgery is progressively becoming the preferred method for gynecological procedures in morbidly obese patients.

Author details

Sharifah Halimah Jaafar[1]*, Iskandar Khalid[2] and Shahridan Mohd Fathil[3]

1 Department of Obstetrics and Gynecology, Gleneagles Hospital Medini Johor, Johor, Malaysia

2 Department of Anaesthesiology and Intensive Care, Hospital Canselor Tuanku Muhriz, UKM, Kuala Lumpur, Malaysia

3 Department of Anesthesiology, Gleneagles Hospital Medini Johor, Johor, Malaysia

*Address all correspondence to: drsharifahclinic@gmail.com

References

[1] Loffer FD, Pent D. Laparoscopy in the obese patient. American Journal of Obstetrics and Gynecology. 1976;**125**:104-108

[2] Holtz G. Laparoscopy in the massively obese female. Obstetrics and Gynecology. 1987;**69**(3 Pt 1):423-424

[3] Capozzi VA, Sozzi G, Gambino G, et al. Laparoscopy versus laparotomy for surgical treatment of obese women with endometrial cancer: A cost-benefit comparative analysis. Molecular and Clinical Oncology. 2019;**11**:335-342

[4] Eltabbakh GH, Piver MS, Hempling RE, Recio FO. Laparoscopic surgery in obese women. Obstetrics and Gynecology. 1999;**94**(5 Pt 1):704-708

[5] Yu CKH, Cutner A, Mould T, Olaitan A. Total laparoscopic hysterectomy as a primary surgical treatment for endometrial cancer in morbidly obese women. BJOG: An International Journal of Obstetrics and Gynaecology. 2005;**112**:115-117

[6] Rooma Sinha G, Swarnasree BR, Madhumathi S. Laparoscopic hysterectomy for large uteri: Outcomes and techniques. Journal of Minimal Access Surgery. 2019;**15**(1):8-13

[7] Blikkendaal MD, Evelyn M, Twijnstra ARH. Hysterectomy in very obese and morbidly obese patients: A systematic review with cumulative analysis of comparative studies. Archives of Gynecology and Obstetrics. 2015;**292**(4):723-738

[8] RollaM,GagliardiML,GiacomantonioL, Cecaroni M, Bruni F, Minelli L, et al. Total laparoscopic hysterectomy of a uterus of 1840 grams: A case report. Acta Bio-Medica. 2009;**80**:282-285

[9] Kondo W, Bourdel N, Marengo F, Botchorishvili R, Pouly JL, Jardon K, et al. Is laparoscopic hysterectomy feasible for uteri larger than 1000 g? European Journal of Obstetrics, Gynecology, and Reproductive Biology. 2011;**158**:76-81

[10] Mullen JT, Moorman DW, Davenport DL. The obesity paradox: Body mass index and outcomes in non bariatric general surgery patients. Annals of Surgery. 2009;**250**(1):166-172. DOI: 10.1097/SLA.0b013e3181a77b1a

[11] Lang LH, Parekh K, Tsui BY, Maze M. Perioperative management of the obese surgical patient. British Medical Bulletin. 2017;**124**:135-155

[12] Ryan NA, Ng VS-M, Sangi-Haghpeykar H. Evaluating mechanical bowel preparation prior to Total laparoscopic hysterectomy. Journal of the Society of Laparoscopic & Robotic Surgeons. 2015;**19**(3):e2015.00035. DOI: 10.4293/JSLS.2015.00035

[13] Apfelbaum JL, Hagberg CA, Caplan RA, et al. Practice guidelines for managing the difficult airway: An updated report by the American Society of anesthesiologists task force on management of the difficult airway. Anesthesiology. 2013;**118**(2):251-270. DOI: 10.1097/ALN.0b013e31827773b2

[14] Juvin P, Lavaut E, Dupont H, Lefevre P, Demetriou M, Dumoulin JL, et al. Difficult tracheal intubation is more common in obese than in lean patients. Anesthesia and Analgesia. 2003;**96**(3):595-600

[15] Piriyapatsom A, Benjasuratwong Y, Vachalathiti R. Comparison of intubation success between direct laryngoscopy and video laryngoscopy in obese patients:

A meta-analysis. Journal of Clinical Anesthesia. 2017;**42**:4-9. DOI: 10.1016/j.jclinane.2017.08.002

[16] Scheib SA, Tanner E 3rd, Green IC, Fader AN. Laparoscopy in the morbidly obese: Physiologic considerations and surgical techniques to optimize success. Journal of Minimally Invasive Gynecology. 2014;**21**:182-195

[17] Zillioux JM, Krupski TL. Patient positioning during minimally invasive surgery: What is the current best practice? Robotic Surgery. 2017;**4**:69-76

[18] Pelosi MA. Alignment of the umbilical axis: An effective maneuver for laparoscopic entry in the obese patient. Obstetrics and Gynecology. 1998;**92**:869-872

[19] Patacchiola F, Palermo P, Kaliakoudas D, Carta A, Mastrocola N, Carta G. The optical trocar in gynecological surgery: Clinical and technical outcomes. Clinical and Experimental Obstetrics & Gynecology. 2012;**39**:519-521. Available from: https://pubmed.ncbi.nlm.nih.gov/23444758/

[20] Louie M, Toubia T, Schiff LD. Considerations for minimally invasive gynecologic surgery in obese patients. Current Opinion in Obstetrics & Gynecology. 2016;**28**:283-289

[21] O'Hanlan KA, Emeney PL, Frank MI, Leila C. Total laparoscopic hysterectomy: Making it safe and successful for obese patients. Journal of the Society of Laparoscopic & Robotic Surgeons. 2021;**25**(2):e2020.00087. DOI: 10.4293/JSLS.2020.00087

[22] Camanni M, Bonino L, Delpiano EM, Migliaretti G, Berchialla P, Deltetto F. Laparoscopy and body mass index: Feasibility and outcome in obese patients treated for gynecologic diseases. Journal of Minimally Invasive Gynecology. 2010;**17**:576-582

[23] Bogani G, Cliby WA, Aletti GD. Impact of morcellation on survival outcomes of patients with unexpected uterine leiomyosarcoma: A systematic review and meta-analysis. Gynecologic Oncology. 2015;**137**(1):167-172. DOI: 10.1016/j.ygyno.2014.11.011

[24] Wang H, Li P, Li X, Gao L, Caihong L, Zhao J, et al. Total laparoscopic hysterectomy in patients with large uteri: Comparison of uterine removal by transvaginal and uterine morcellation approaches. BioMed Research International. 2016;**2016**:8784601. DOI: 10.1155/2016/8784601

Chapter 4

Adhesiolysis during Hysterectomy

Gatot Purwoto and Kartiwa Hadi Nuryanto

Abstract

Hysterectomy sometimes is not as simple as removing the uterus. The most challenging condition before definitive hysterectomy is mostly an adhesion with various grade of severity and need a careful approach to prevent surrounding organ injury. Adhesions can be a significant source of morbidity in patients and provide a thorough overview of the etiology, pathophysiology, and clinical consequences. The authors provide a step-by-step approach including preoperative preparation, surgical techniques, and postoperative management. This chapter also explains the prevention of adhesions and the use of adhesion barriers. With contributions from leading experts in the field, it seems to be an essential resource for any surgeon seeking to optimize patient outcomes in laparotomy. This comprehensive guide might be used by surgeons to improve their understanding and technical skills in dealing with adhesions during laparotomy.

Keywords: adhesiolysis, hysterectomy, surgical techniques, adhesion, incision

1. Introduction

Fibrous bands of scar tissue are defined as abdominal adhesion, which spans into two or more intra-abdominal organs, or sometimes that inner abdominal wall arises after abdominal surgery. Adhesions might also form as a result of inflammatory abdominal conditions without prior abdominal surgery or as a sequel to abdomino-pelvic radiation [1, 2]. Postoperative adhesions are a natural consequence of surgical tissue trauma and healing. Although the majority of patients with intra-abdominal adhesions remain asymptomatic, a clinically significant subset of patients will develop "adhesive disease," a symptomatic state ranging from mild and/or vague to highly distressing and even life-threatening symptoms [2].

2. Etiology

Adhesions are the result of tissue injury, likely to occur by the injury of an incision, electrocoagulation trauma and sutures, infection, or by foreign bodies damaging the parietal and visceral peritoneum, which reacts forming abundant aberrant peritoneal healing and scars [1, 3]. Ischemia has been proposed as the most important injury that leads to adhesion development. Another possible underlying mechanism may be a deficient, suppressed, or overwhelmed natural immune system [1].

The most common location of adhesion is within the abdominal cavity and the pelvis. Abdominal adhesions are a common complication of surgery. The most common is in the small intestinal. Pelvic adhesions may involve any organ, such as the uterus, ovaries, fallopian tubes, or bladder, and usually occur after surgery. Pelvic inflammatory disease (PID) results from an infection that frequently leads to adhesions within the fallopian tubes. Fallopian adhesions can lead to infertility and increased incidence of ectopic pregnancy. Endometriosis may also cause pelvic adhesions.

3. Pathophysiology

Adhesion formation has three steps;: (A) inhibition of extracellular matrix degradation system and fibrinolytic (B) induction of an inflammatory response involving cytokine production and transforming growth factor-β (TGF-β); and (C) induction of tissue hypoxia, leading to increase in expression of vascular endothelial growth factor (VEGF). As adhesions mature their cell population changes from days one to three, cells are mainly polymorphonuclear cells (PMN) leukocytes, whereas between days five and seven fibroblasts predominate [4]. Factors that have been identified include those important for the regulation of inflammatory and immune responses, tissue remodeling, and angiogenesis.

Cellular insult results in an outpouring of fibrin and subsequent fibrinolysis. The insult causes hypoxia and the release of reactive oxygen species (ROS), which lead to inflammation and activation of the coagulation cascade. This increases the production of thrombin, which is a key activator of fibrin [4, 5]. Fibrin production and fibrinolysis are part of the physiologic process; if the balance between fibrin production and fibrinolysis becomes compromised pathological adhesion formation occurs [4].

Deposition of fibrin monomers (red and white blood cells, macrophages, platelets, and tissue exudates) develops a polymeric matrix within which fibroblasts can adhere and produce components of extracellular matrix (ECM), setting the stage for mature adhesion formation [3–5]. A major determinant of the persistence of the fibrinous mass is the degree of plasminogen activator activity (PAA). PAA, which can be considered to be represented by the ratio of tissue plasminogen activator (tPA) to its inhibitor, plasminogen activator inhibitor 1 (PAI-1), resides in both the mesothelial cells and the underlying fibroblasts [5]. Plasminogen activator inhibitors (PAIs) can prevent PAs from activating plasmin, leading to compromised fibrinolytic activity [6].

Then proliferating fibroblasts invade and keep extracellular matrix material including collagen and also have contributed to the formation of adhesion. And next step is after elicitation of angiogenesis factor, for example vascular endothelial growth factor (VEGF). Imbalances in any of these could potentially contribute to adhesion development [1].

It has been shown that fibroblasts derived from tissue adhesions have a different phenotype (myofibroblasts) when compared to normal fibroblasts found in peritoneal tissue. Transformation of the phenotype has been associated with tissue hypoxia, whereas fibroblast adhesions determine increased mRNA expression of fibronectin, collagen I, metalloproteinase-1, Tissue Growth Factor TGF-beta1, Tissue Inhibitors of Metalloproteinases (TIMP-1), Cyclooxygenase-2 (COX-2), and IL-10. All of these proteins support the formation of adhesion action at different times [3, 7].

An enzyme that regulates the inflammatory process of angiogenesis in the formation of postoperative adhesions is COX-2. In the presence of tissue hypoxia and/or fibroblast adhesion, COX-2 expression is increased. While the formation of dense postoperative adhesions, the fibrinolytic system has an important role in converting plasminogen to plasmin. The conversion is determined by the tissue Plasminogen Activator (tPA) and activator-type urokinase (uPA), both are expressed by the complex of the endothelial and mesothelial cells, macrophages, and fibroblasts. The tPA has been shown to be responsible for the plasminogen activation and fibrin degradation, whereas uPA plays a role during tissue remodeling [1, 3].

The process of adhesion formation might be regarded as an ischemic disease. Under hypoxic conditions, metabolic enzymes are regulated via hypoxic responsive elements by the hypoxia-inducible factor 1 (HIF-1) [8]. Molecular pathways involved in fibrinolysis inhibition, inflammation, and tissue hypoxia crosstalk and potentiate the effect of each. The principal molecular aberrations included the reduction of tissue plasminogen activator (tPA) and up-regulation of TGF-β1 and HIF-1α [1].

4. Clinical consequences of adhesion formation

Small bowel obstruction, infertility, and chronic abdominal pain are generally mentioned as the main clinical consequences formation of adhesion [9]. The most important risk of adhesion formation is infertility, abdominal or pelvic pain, obstruction of the bowel, and injury to intra-abdominal structure on another or next surgeries. Imaging tools such as the visceral slide test have been used to determine the presence of periumbilical adhesions before laparoscopy. However, there is no other method for identifying preoperative adhesions and only direct visualization on surgery that accurately identify and measure postoperative adhesion, though periumbilical adhesions could be detected by ultrasonography [10, 11].

The most common cause of postoperative small-bowel obstruction is adhesions [12]. The incidence of small bowel obstruction is 2–3 percent in the first year after surgery in all patients who undergo abdominal or pelvic surgery [13]. The risk of adhesive small bowel obstruction depends on the anatomical location of surgery, the breadth of surgery, and peritoneal injury [13, 14]. And risk varies in abdominal wall surgery from 0.5 percent; 1.2 percent after upper gastrointestinal surgery to 3.2 percent in lower gastrointestinal surgery and 4.2 percent in pediatric surgery [13].

Infertility and adhesions may affect fertility adversely by distorting adnexal anatomy and interfering with gamete and embryo transport. Among infertile women with unexplained infertility diagnosed with adnexal adhesions by laparoscopy, the pregnancy rates were 32 percent at 12 months after subsequent adhesiolysis by laparotomy and 45 percent at 24 months compared with 11 percent at 12 months and 16 percent at 24 months in untreated women [15].

In another study of 198 patients after lower gastrointestinal tract surgery for adhesive small bowel obstruction, 40 percent of patients developed chronic abdominal pain. In four studies following patients with chronic postoperative pain after previous surgery, adhesions were identified as the most likely cause of pain during diagnostic laparoscopy in 57 percent of patients [13]. The relationship between adhesions and pelvic pain is unclear. Between the extent of adhesions and the severity of pain, there is no relationship. In some cases, adhesions may cause visceral pain with impairing organ immobility. A study of patients with chronic pelvic pain randomized to laparotomy with adhesiolysis or laparotomy only, found adhesiolysis was effective for those who had dense adhesions involving the bowel.

5. Adhesiolysis technique

5.1 Step-by-step approach

5.1.1 Preoperative evaluation

Preoperative evaluation should be taken from patient's general medical condition and prior surgical history, especially abdominal surgery. The evaluation could be prepared by understanding patient's medical history and performing a complete physical examination. Careful attention can substantiate the suspicion of adhesions including medical history, current medications, allergies to medications, food, or environmental agents, previous surgical procedures, family history, and others. Repeated laparotomies, including Cesarean sections (C-sections), maybe a risk factor for intra-abdominal adhesion. Informed consent is taken after preoperative discussion which includes a description of the surgical procedure and its expected outcomes and risks like adhesion. This is the basis for obtaining signed informed consent [16, 17]. Intra-abdominal adhesions are diagnosed intra-operatively. Evidence points of adhesions may be yielded by high-resolution ultrasonography and functional MRI; both could detect limited movement relative. To one another of organs joined by adhesions [17].

5.1.2 Surgical techniques

Adhesiolysis is an inadvertent injury while performing surgery. Injuries when adhesiolysis are made in the bowel most frequently, which classified as bellowing injury [18]:

- Injury of seromuscular, an injury to the visceral peritoneum or serosa layer and smooth muscle layer of the bowel, and usually the bowel lumen or leakage of bowel contents is not visible

- Enterotomy is a full-thickness injury to the bowel

- Delayed diagnosed perforation, and unrecognized bowel injuries that were made during surgery.

Steps in abdominal hysterectomy with enterolysis:

5.1.2.1 Skin incision

The incision is carried down through the subcutaneous tissue and fascia, and so does the peritoneum.

5.1.2.2 Exploration of abdominal

Upper abdomen and pelvis are systematically explored. The liver, stomach, gallbladder, large and small intestines, kidneys, and pelvic and para-aortic lymph nodes should be examined and palpated. We need to give attention to bilateral ovaries

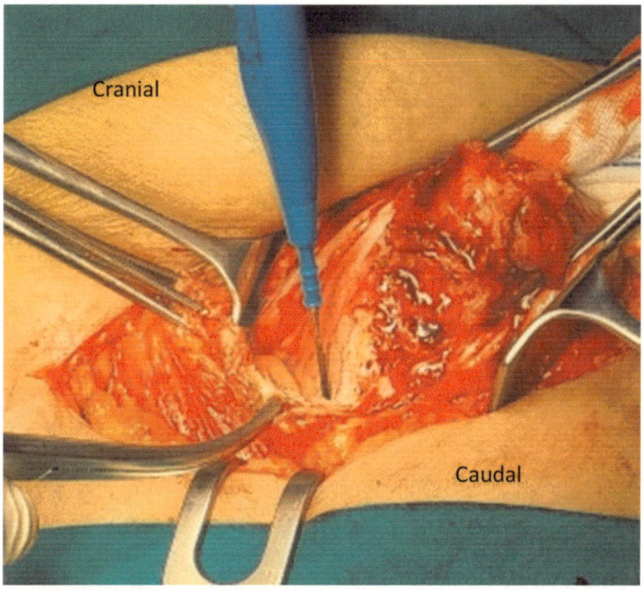

Figure 1.
Adhesiolysis abdominal wall and uterus in previous surgical scar.

uterus, uterus and fallopian tubes, ligaments, bladder, and rectosigmoid colon for any adhesions between these organs which should be evaluated carefully.

5.1.2.3 Retraction of wound

Surgeons should choose an appropriate retractor for each patient. There were a variety of retractors designed for abdominal and pelvic surgery (**Figure 1**).

5.1.2.4 Transection of infundibulo-pelvic ligament, fallopian tube, and utero-ovarian ligament

In the retroperitoneal space, the ureter may be identified. When we need to preserve the ovaries, the utero-ovarian ligament and fallopian tubes are grasped with forceps, cut, and suture ligated. Otherwise, the ovaries tend to be removed, and the window of peritoneal opening is enlarged sufficiently to expose the ovarian vessels inside the infundibulopelvic ligament, uterine artery, and ureter. The infundibulopelvic ligament is grasped with forceps, cut, and suture ligated. The ovarian vessels are ligated. The connective tissue around the cardinal ligament is removed, and the posterior leaf of the broad ligament is divided inferiorly toward the uterosacral ligament to aid in uterine mobilization (**Figures 2** and **3**).

5.1.2.5 Round ligament ligation

Placing clamps on the broad ligament to elevate the uterus, providing traction and securing the field of view. The round ligament was then grasped with forceps at its proximal and distal portions. Transected using suture ligation. Broad ligament is incised to separate the anterior and posterior leaves. These steps are applied on the

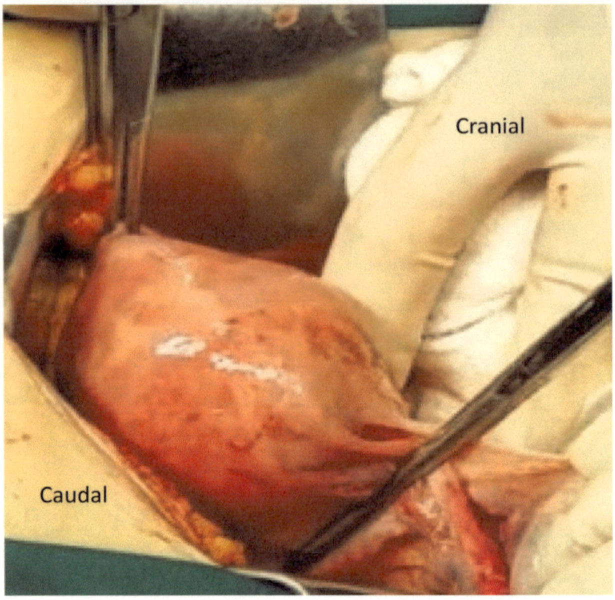

Figure 2.
Clamping of utero-ovarian ligament (round ligament, fallopian tube, ovarian-proprium ligament).

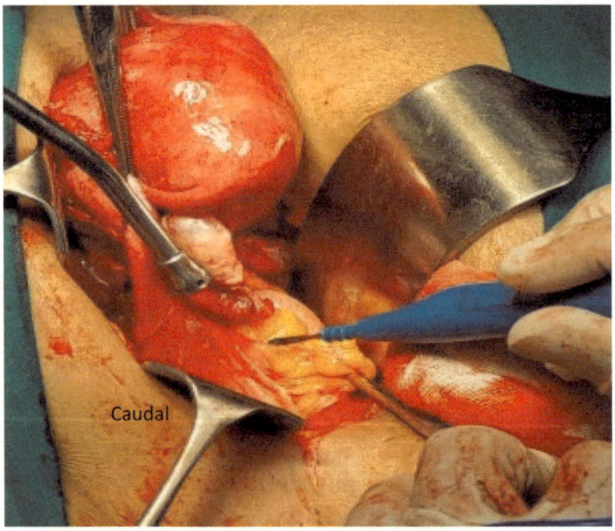

Figure 3.
Adhesiolysis left adnexa and rectum.

contralateral side. The anterior leaf of the broad ligament is then incised using an electrical scalpel along the vesicouterine fold, separating the bladder from lower uterine segment (**Figures 4–6**).

5.1.2.6 Release adhesion to surrounding organs

Lysis of adhesions can be performed as a part of the various procedures in abdominal cavity. Adhesiolysis is releasing adhesions either by blunt or sharp dissection

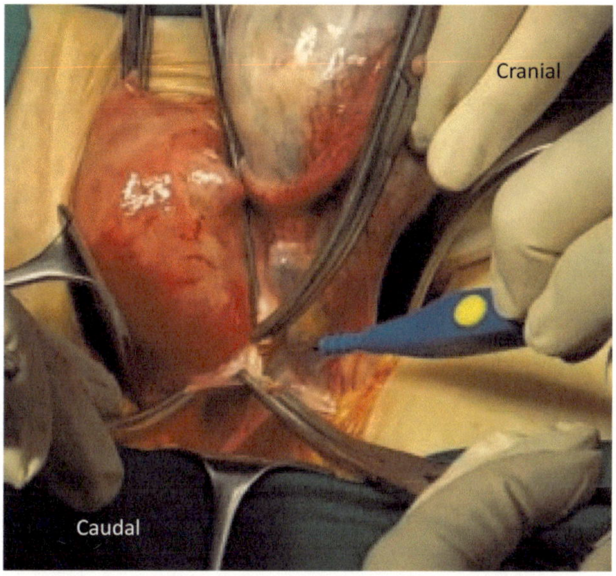

Figure 4.
Clamp and cut left round ligament. The round ligament is grasped with forceps at its proximal and distal portion and transected.

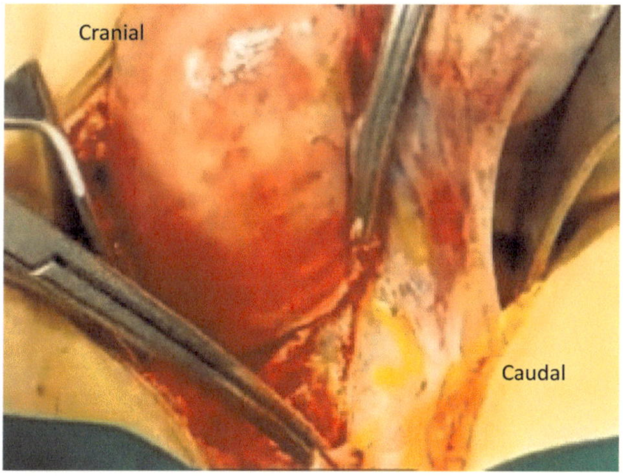

Figure 5.
Opening retroperitoneal space to identify ureter.

during surgery. The standard method of removing adhesions using "blunt dissection" is to pull adhesions apart with gentle traction during surgery. The main principles of adhesion prevention and complications are minimizing surgical trauma and could use adjuvants to reduce adhesion formation. Adhesiolysis can be done during laparoscopy or open laparotomy. In case of severe and extensive adhesion would be safer with open laparotomy. Severe adhesion between uterus and bowel during open laparotomy (**Figures 7–9**).

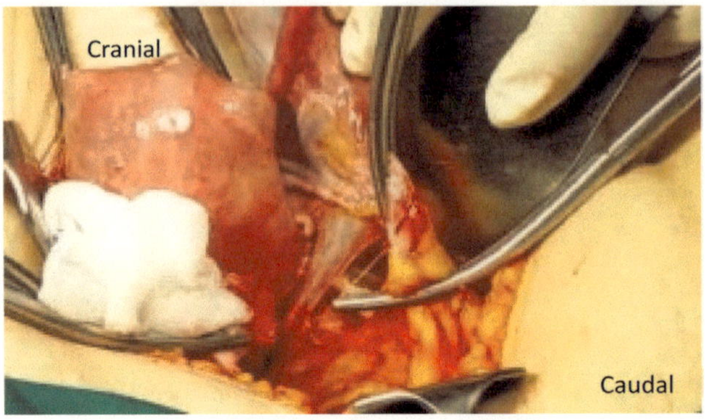

Figure 6.
Clamp and cut infundibulo-pelvic ligament after identified ureter.

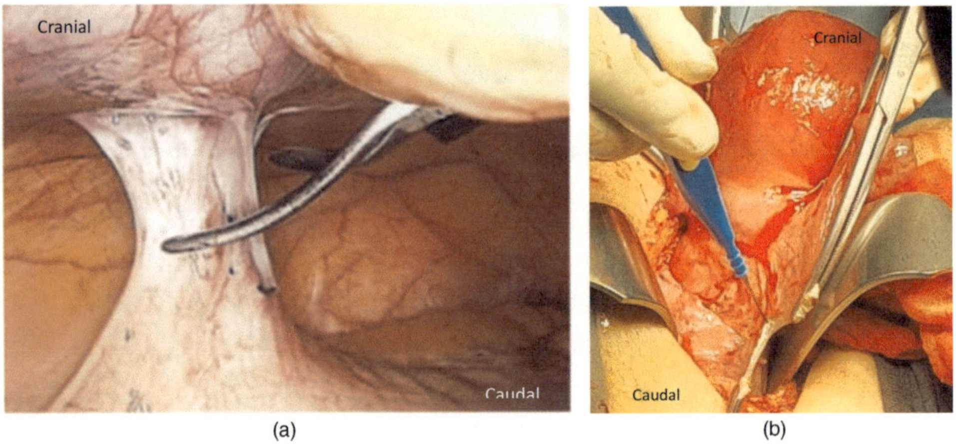

Figure 7.
(a) Fibrin adhesiolysis in laparoscopy. (b) Adhesiolysis in open laparotomy.

5.1.2.7 Cardinal ligament ligation

Two curved forceps at the level of the internal os of the cervix are dissected and clamp the uterine artery and vein. The vessels are cut and suture ligated. Then the remaining cardinal ligament is clamped, cut, and suture ligated. These steps are repeated two or three times until reach the level of the cervicovaginal junction. The bladder and rectum are inspected to be sure they are clear of the surgical specimen. At this point, the anterior and posterior vaginal walls are exposed (**Figure 10**).

5.1.2.8 Uterus removal

The uterus is placed on the traction of cephalad direction and vaginalis portion of the cervix is palpated. Incision is made in the vaginal wall, beneath the cervicovaginal junction, using an electrical scalpel. Then the uterus is removed (**Figure 11**).

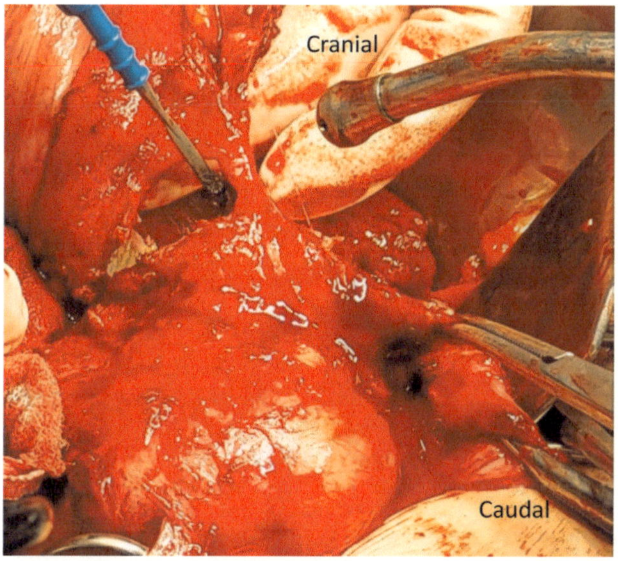

Figure 8.
Adhesiolysis posterior part of uterus and anterior part of rectum.

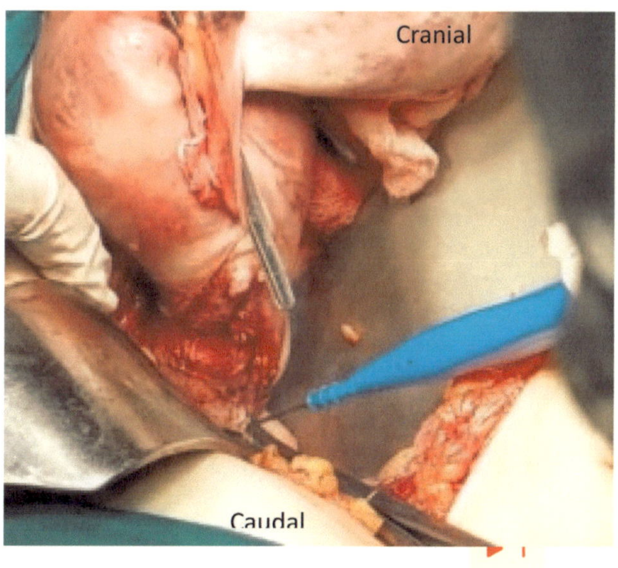

Figure 9.
Clamp and cut uterine artery and vein.

5.1.2.9 Closure of the vaginal cuff

Make sure the bladder and rectum should be clearly seen in the operative field, and the vaginal cuff is cross-clamped using forceps to achieve hemostasis and provide traction. The vaginal cuff is typically closed by suturing (**Figure 12**).

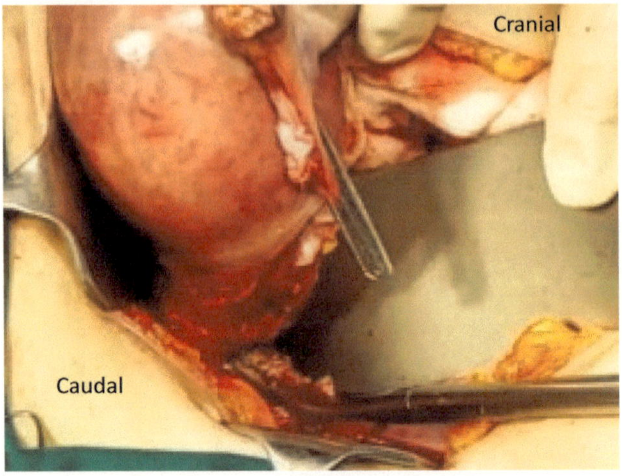

Figure 10.
Clamp and cut cardinal and uterosacral ligament.

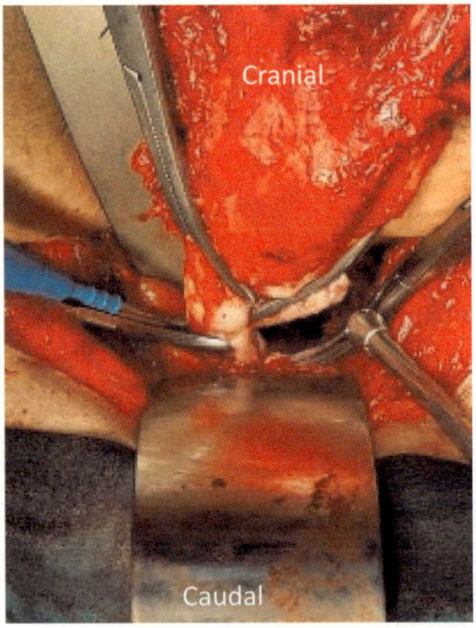

Figure 11.
Cutting uterus at the level of fornix.

5.1.2.10 Irrigation and hemostasis

The pelvis is irrigated with warm saline. We should ensure carefully the vascular pedicles for complete hemostasis. Suture ligation or electrocautery is used to control bleeding in small areas. The bladder, ureter, and rectosigmoid colon should be checked to confirm that they are intact. Adhesion formation could be prevented by anti-adhesive material.

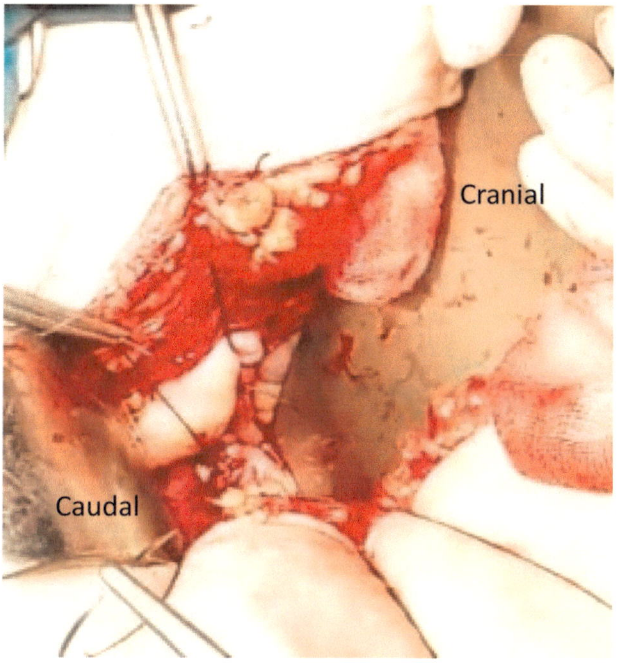

Figure 12.
Vaginal stump closure with no. 1 PGA.

5.1.2.11 Fascia and skin closure

Interrupted or continuous suturing could be used for closing the fascia. For hemostasis, subcutaneous tissue should be irrigated and inspected carefully. The wound disruption risk seems to be decreased with subcutaneous fat layer closure or with continuous low-pressure suction for draining subcutaneous hemorrhage or exudate in obese women. Skin closure is performed using either staples or subcuticular sutures with adhesive tape.

5.1.3 Postoperative management

Postoperative care is important for general management and wound management. Prophylactic antibiotics and suction drainage are the key points for wound healing. Wound dehiscence and infection should be managed by good wound bed preparation.

6. The prevention of adhesions and the use of adhesion barriers

Adhesion barriers are adjuvants for peritoneal administration that can reduce adhesion formation [18]. Anti-adhesive material used to prevent adhesion formation, especially in patients who already have intraperitoneal adhesions from previous surgery, pelvic inflammatory disease, or endometriosis [16]. There are several forms of adhesion barriers: solid membranes, gels, and liquids. Adhesion barrier act as a spacer that separates injured surfaces of the peritoneum, allowing these surfaces to heal without forming fibrinous attachment, which eventually leads to adhesions. Barriers should be inert to the human immune system and be slowly degradable. Adhesion barriers might also be used to prevent recurrence after surgical treatment. The most common applied adhesion barriers and their impact on adhesion formation are described below [8]:

1. Hyaluronate carboxymethylcellulose adhesion barrier can reduce the incidence of reoperations for adhesive small bowel obstruction.

2. Oxidized regenerated cellulose, a solid barrier most suitable for open surgery and reduces incidence of adhesion formation.

3. Icodextrin, a liquid barrier which easy to apply in both open and laparoscopic surgery.

4. Polyethylene glycol, a gel barrier which easy to apply in both open and laparoscopic surgery.

Author details

Gatot Purwoto* and Kartiwa Hadi Nuryanto
University of Indonesia – Cipto Mangunkusumo Hospital, Jakarta, Indonesia

*Address all correspondence to: gatotpurwoto@gmail.com

References

[1] Buțureanu SA, Buțureanu TAS. Pathophysiology of adhesions. Chirurgia (Romania). 2014;**109**(3):293-298

[2] Tabibian N, Swehli E, Boyd A, Umbreen A, Tabibian JH. Abdominal adhesions: A practical review of an often overlooked entity. Annals of Medicine and Surgery. 2017;**15**:9-13

[3] Guzmán-Valdivia-Gómez G, Tena-Betancourt E, De Alva-Coria PM. Postoperative abdominal adhesions: Pathogenesis and current preventive techniques. Cirugia y Cirujanos. 2019; **87**(6):698-703

[4] Hassanabad AF, Zarzycki AN, Jeon K, Deniset JF, Fedak PWM. Post-operative adhesions: A comprehensive review of mechanisms. Biomedicine. 2021;**9**(8): 1-19

[5] Awonuga AO, Belotte J, Abuanzeh S, Fletcher NM, Diamond MPSG. Advances in the pathogenesis of adhesion development: The role of oxidative stress. Reproductive Sciences. 2012; **21**(7):823-836

[6] Palta S, Saroa R, Palta A. Overview of the coagulation system. Indian Journal of Anaesthesia. 2014;**58**(5):515-523

[7] Chen YT, Chang YT, Pan SY, Chou YH, Chang FC, Yeh PY, et al. Lineage tracing reveals distinctive fates for mesothelial cells and submesothelial fibroblasts during peritoneal injury. Journal of the American Society of Nephrology. 2014;**25**(12):2847-2858

[8] Wallwiener M, Wallwiener CW, Molinas R, Rajab TK, Brucker SY, Kraemer B, et al. Intraabdominal adhesion formation is associated with differential mRNA expression of metabolic genes PDHb and SDHa. Archives of Gynecology and Obstetrics. 2012;**286**(3):683-686

[9] Zwanenburg ES, Wisselink DD, Klaver CEL, Brandt ARM, Bremers AJA, Burger JWA, et al. Adhesion formation after surgery for locally advanced colonic cancer in the COLOPEC trial. British Journal of Surgery. 2022;**109**(4): 315-318

[10] Nezhat CH, Dun EC, Katz A, Wieser FA. Office visceral slide test compared with two perioperative tests for predicting periumbilical adhesions. Obstetrics and Gynecology. 2014;**123**(5): 1049-1056

[11] Lee M, Kim HS, Chung HH, Kim JW, Park NH, Song YS. Prediction of intra-abdominal adhesions using the visceral slide test: A prospective observational study. European Journal of Obstetrics and Gynecology and Reproductive Biology. 2017;**213**:22-25

[12] Krielen P, Stommel WJ, ten Broek PG, van Goor H. Adhesive small bowel obstruction in the minimally invasive era. In: Garbuzenko DV, editor. Intestinal Obstructions. Russia; 2020. p. 94

[13] Richard PG, Issa Y, Van Santbrink EJP, Bouvy ND, Kruitwagen RFPM, Jeekel J, et al. Burden of adhesions in abdominal and pelvic surgery: Systematic review and met-analysis. BMJ (Online). 2013;**347**(7929): 1-15

[14] Coccolini F, Ansaloni L, Manfredi R, Campanati L, Poiasina E, Bertoli P, et al. Peritoneal adhesion index (PAI): Proposal of a score for the "ignored iceberg" of medicine and surgery. World Journal of Emergency Surgery. 2013; **8**(1):1-5

[15] Penzias A, Bendikson K, Falcone T, Gitlin S, Gracia C, Hansen K, et al. Postoperative adhesions in gynecologic surgery: A committee opinion. Fertility and Sterility. 2019;**112**(3):458-463

[16] Editor M. Comprehensive Gynecology and Obstetrics [Internet]. Available from: http://www.springer.com/series/13621

[17] Brüggmann D, Tchartchian G, Wallwiener M, Münstedt K, Tinneberg HR, Hackethal A. Intraabdominale adhäsionen - Definition, entstehung, bedeutung in der operativen medizin und möglichkeiten der reduktion. Deutsches Arzteblatt. 2010;**107**:769-775

[18] ten Broek RPG, Krielen P, Di Saverio S, Coccolini F, Biffl WL, Ansaloni L, et al. Bologna guidelines for diagnosis and management of adhesive small bowel obstruction (ASBO): 2017 update of the evidence-based guidelines from the world society of emergency surgery ASBO working group. World Journal of Emergency Surgery. 2018;**13**

Section 3

Vaginal Birth after Cesarean

Chapter 5

Experience of Having a Vaginal Birth after Cesarean Section in Order to Prevent Postpartum Complication Using Narrative Review

Eman Alshawish

Abstract

Vaginal birth after cesarean (VBAC) is defined as a vaginal delivery by a woman who has had a previous cesarean delivery. Vaginal birth can lead to quicker post birth recovery, less operative trauma, shorter length of hospital stays, and improved feelings of wellness. It is well-known that C-section now, hysterectomy complications later. This review aims to explore the existing research on VBAC in order to prevent postpartum complication. This review commences with the exploration of women's attitudes around VBAC, education and decision on their mode of birth. Eight main themes were: Women's attitudes and views of VBAC; VBAC education and decision-making programs; previous VBAC; maternal morbidity and mortality; short inter-pregnancy interval; induction of labor; neonatal morbidity and mortality; and birth trauma. Evidence shows that midwives have a positive influence on VBAC rates without an increase in maternal or neonatal morbidity. Review revealed the limited comprehension and awareness regarding the factors influencing women's decision to opt VBAC, and the viewpoints held by midwives. The recommendation is to increase the number of VBAC by emphasizing on midwifery role, continuity of care, education program, and conducting more research.

Keywords: vaginal birth after cesarean section (VBAC), cesarean section (CS), prevent postpartum complication, midwife, experience

1. Introduction

Vaginal birth after cesarean (VBAC) is defined as a vaginal delivery by a woman who has had a previous cesarean delivery [1]. When women receive support to undergo a VBAC, numerous advantages arise for the women themselves, their families, and society as a whole. Opting for a vaginal birth can result in swifter post-birth recovery, reduced surgical trauma, shorter hospital stays, and enhanced overall well-being, encompassing physical and psychological aspects for women [2]. VBAC is associated with lower maternal mortality and less overall morbidity for mothers and babies [3]. It is well-known that C-section now, hysterectomy complications later. In cases where women had previously delivered through cesarean section, the likelihood of encountering surgical complications increased during hysterectomy procedures. According to a comprehensive Danish cohort study that looked back at past records, women with a history of C-section had elevated rates of reoperation within 30 days and experienced more perioperative and postoperative complications when undergoing a benign hysterectomy compared to women who had delivered vaginally [4].

This review aims to explore the existing research on VBAC to provide a background and purpose to this paper. The review encompassed a range of research methodologies, including qualitative and quantitative approaches. It begins by examining women's attitudes and perspectives toward VBAC, along with investigating VBAC education and the decision-making process for choosing the mode of birth. The study identifies various factors that contribute to achieving a VBAC, which are further categorized into sub-themes. Furthermore, the review delves into the morbidity and mortality risks associated with cesarean sections, as well as comparative studies comparing the risks and outcomes of VBAC versus cesarean deliveries. Additionally, the review places emphasis on the outcomes of VBAC births that occur outside of hospitals, the management of VBAC within hospital settings, and the existing research on birth trauma. Within the topic of birth trauma, the review explores women's emotional experiences related to their previous traumatic births, including some that involved cesarean sections, and also highlights the potential healing effects of a positive subsequent birth.

2. Literature review method

A search of the following databases was undertaken: CINAHL, Medline, Scopus, PubMed, and Cochrane. Papers published in the last 10 years were included to ensure key papers were identified. The study utilized specific keywords such as cesarean, VBAC, vaginal birth after cesarean, and childbirth. To maintain objectivity, opinion pieces and anecdotal articles were excluded. Additional papers were discovered by examining the reference lists of the included studies, leading to a snowball effect in the search process. A total of 45 studies were carefully reviewed and contributed to the construction of this literature review.

2.1 Women's attitudes and views of VBAC

The literature review begins by examining and analyzing the existing research regarding women's attitudes and perspectives toward VBAC, as it is one of the primary areas of focus for this review. While the review concentrates on the experiences of women who undergo VBAC, there is currently a lack of research that specifically addresses the experiences of this particular group. Nevertheless, there are research papers available that explore the attitudes and views of women who choose to have a VBAC.

A total of four qualitative studies and one quantitative study were identified, all of which delve into women's attitudes and experiences regarding VBAC. Among these studies, three focused on the perceptions and experiences of women who planned to have a VBAC in a hospital setting, while one specifically explored the experiences of women who opted for a water VBAC in a midwife-led unit [5]. A common thread observed across these studies was the emphasis on informed choice, variations in postpartum recovery, and factors influencing the bonding process [6–9]. The women actively attempted to minimize the medicalization of childbirth by limiting medical staff input. Opting for Water VBAC was a means of avoiding the 'cascade of obstetric interventions [5].

Women observed variations in the manner in which healthcare providers either positively encouraged or negatively impacted their choice to pursue a VBAC. For some women, when healthcare providers presented options and actively involved them in the decision-making process, they felt a sense of trust toward their healthcare provider [9]. Other women found that the healthcare provider did not give sufficient information [5] and implied VBAC was very risky, which resulted in the women feeling bullied into following the staff recommendations and later made to feel guilty if anything was to go wrong [8]. Fenwick et al. [6] also reported the positive effect of family and friends' attitudes toward VBAC, the effect of reflection on the previous cesarean, as well as the benefit of VBAC to the health of the baby.

Other quantitative research reflex attitude of women reports the effect of reflection on the previous cesarean as well as the benefit of VBAC to see vaginal delivery as the natural method of childbirth, and even more appealing to them is the faster recovery after a vaginal delivery as compared to CS [10].

In a qualitative study in Cyprus that adopted phenomenological study, participants described their previous experience of CS as traumatic in contrast to vaginal birth and their need of evidence-based information, guidelines of birthing options, good preparation, and personalized care [7].

In a study conducted by Dahlen and Homer [11], discussions about VBAC on international blog sites were explored. The primary theme that emerged was labeled as 'mother birth/childbirth'. Within the 'mother birth' framework, women expressed the belief that a mother's health and well-being were crucial for the well-being of the baby, and they considered the birth experience to be significant in achieving this. These women balanced their own needs with those of the baby and were more inclined to choose a VBAC. On the other hand, the 'childbirth' framework described women who prioritized the needs of the baby over their own and opted for what they perceived to be the less risky option, namely, elective cesarean. Other themes that emerged in line with previous research included the importance of choice, fear of giving birth, and perceptions of body failure [11].

2.2 VBAC education and decision-making programs

A total of nine studies examined in the decision-making process of women in choosing between aiming for a VBAC or opting for a repeat elective cesarean section. Among these studies, five included an educational program as part of their investigation, focusing on understanding how such programs might impact decision-making and outcomes [12–16]. This study explored the effect of a variety of educational programs on women's decision making and VBAC outcomes.

The women stated that they need information about VBAC from supportive clinicians, but they also asked for information from other women with experiences of VBAC; the women prefer calm surroundings during birth and clinicians who are confident with VBAC [17, 18]. Other studies that Bako et al. conducted found differences in the way healthcare providers either positively supported or negatively influenced their decision to pursue a VBAC. Certain women discovered that by receiving counseling from healthcare providers during pregnancy, along with the implementation of public education campaigns to enable informed decision-making, they were able to develop trust in their healthcare providers. This trust will help them to take their decision [10].

Three studies explored the effect of a variety of educational programs on women's decision-making and VBAC outcomes. These included a face-to-face education program versus a pamphlet [13], a 90 minute computer-based information resource [16], and an information program covering issues such as complications for the mother and baby compared with a decision analysis program [15]. The effectiveness of the aforementioned programs showed varying results, potentially influenced by a bias in the program content. For instance, Wang et al. [16], despite conducting a small study, observed a positive shift in attitude and increased knowledge among participants after the intervention. This resulted in an increase in the number of women planning to have a VBAC, with the count rising from six to nine and, ultimately, eight of them successfully achieving a VBAC. The program had a positive orientation toward VBAC and incorporated the personal experiences of other women who had undergone VBAC.

However, in the study done by Frost et al. that included interviews with 30 of the women from the Diamond trial, key themes were: role of decision aids in reducing decisional conflict and uncertainty during the pregnancy; impact of decision aids on knowledge and anxiety; the relationship between prior preferences, decisions, and actual outcome; and the mediating role of decision aids. It was found that some of the women's concerns about both the decision analysis tool and the information provision for VBAC [14]. They should be relevant to their individual needs. One study found that women who scored high on motivation for vaginal birth were more likely to have a VBAC, regardless of education style [13].

2.3 Previous VBAC

According to Mercer et al. [19], women who had previously experienced a VBAC were more inclined to have a vaginal birth in subsequent pregnancies. The study revealed that for women without a prior VBAC, the rate of VBAC was 63.3%. However, if they had one previous VBAC, the rate increased to 87.6%, and for those with two or more previous VBACs, the rate further rose to 90.9% [19]. Interestingly, women who had a history of two or more VBACs also tended to have undergone multiple cesarean sections; a number of factors are associated with VBAC, including previous vaginal birth, particularly previous VBAC, being the single best predictor for VBAC and is associated with an approximately 87–90% planned VBAC rate [20, 21].

2.4 Maternal morbidity & mortality in cesarean versus planned VBAC

In this section, the literature review will focus on large multicenter studies that have investigated the disparities in maternal morbidity and mortality among women with a previous cesarean section and the various modes of birth for subsequent deliveries. These studies have highlighted specific outcomes related to maternal morbidities, such as endometritis, increased bleeding necessitating blood transfusion, and operative injuries, in the context of planned VBAC compared to elective cesarean sections [22–25]. However, when examining the data that identifies the mode of birth within the planned VBAC group, it becomes evident that the heightened morbidities are primarily attributable to emergency cesarean sections. For instance, in the study by Landon et al. [24] that focused on planned VBACs resulting in cesarean sections, the rate of endometritis was 7.7% compared to 1.2% for vaginal births and 1.8% for elective cesarean sections. Similarly, the need for a blood transfusion when a VBAC was unsuccessful was 3.2%, compared to 1.2% for successful VBACs and 1.0% for elective cesarean sections [24].

Factors that increase uterine rupture rate Fear of uterine rupture is one of the key deterrents for VBAC [26]. The uterine rupture rate varies in different studies, from 0.1% to 2.7% [23, 24, 27, 28]. An Australian study found the uterine rupture rate was 0.2% [22].

Several studies have examined the factors associated with increased rates of uterine rupture in women with a history of previous cesarean sections. Two specific factors have been identified: the interval between the cesarean section and subsequent pregnancy (known as the inter-pregnancy interval) and the use of pharmacological agents to induce labor. These factors have been investigated in studies conducted by Smith et al. [29], Buhimschi et al. [30], Stamilio et al. [28], Fitzpatrick et al. [31], Stock et al. [32], and Palatnik and Grobman [33].

A systematic review study by Wu et al. [34] that included 94 studies found the most factors affecting the success of VBAC were diabetes, hypertensive disorders complicating pregnancy, Bishop score, labor induction, macrosomia, age, obesity, previous vaginal birth, and the indications for the previous CS. The midwife should take into her consideration these factors to increase success of VBAC. Also, a complete obstetric history is important for a safe VBAC [35].

2.5 Short inter-pregnancy interval

Stamilio et al. [28] conducted a study focusing on the influence of short pregnancy intervals. The findings indicate that women with a short inter-pregnancy period, defined as the time between the birth of one child and the conception of the next pregnancy, have a higher rate of uterine rupture at 2.7% compared to a rate of 0.9% for women with an interval of more than 6 months. However, the rate of successful VBAC did not differ significantly, remaining at 77%. One study that focused on the reported cases of women who had experienced a uterine rupture found rupture rates increased with a short inter-pregnancy interval of less than 12 months and where induction/augmentation occurred [31]. Royal College of Obstetricians and Gynecologists [36] guidelines state a period of less than 18 months since the previous cesarean is a contraindication to VBAC.

2.6 Induction of labor

Studies have looked at the impact of using pharmaceutical techniques for induction or augmentation of labor (IOL) on the incidence rate of uterine rupture in women trying a VBAC. The highest rate of uterine rupture tends to occur following a multi-pharmacological use of prostaglandin gel and oxytocin [29, 30, 32, 33]. Alternatives to pharmacological IOL have been explored in a study on serial membrane sweeping [37]. With 108 participants in the sweeping group and 105 in the control group, the sample size was small. There was no difference in the primary outcomes of labor induction or the frequency of repeat cesarean deliveries, and there were no uterine ruptures during the treatment, which involved either weekly membrane sweeping or weekly vaginal inspections [37]. A recent study [38] has reported no differences in VBAC success rates or neonatal and maternal outcomes for women who had one or more prior cesareans and used pharmacological induction of labor techniques.

Women who had continuity of care (CoC) with a midwife were more likely to feel in control of their decision-making and believe their healthcare provider supported their decision to have a VBAC, according to the Australian VBAC survey by Keedle et al. [39].

Women who underwent CoC with a midwife were more likely to be active during labor, to experience submersion in water, and to give delivery in an upright position.

2.7 Neonatal morbidity and mortality

The large studies that compared the outcomes of VBAC verses elective cesarean also included neonatal morbidity and mortality [22, 24]. One study found an increase in the rate of antepartum stillbirth in the planned VBAC cohort (0.6%) compared with the elective cesarean group (0.2%) [22]. The authors did identify that these numbers included babies with known congenital malformations and women experiencing fetal death in utero who were encouraged to have a VBAC rather than a cesarean. Neonatals born via vaginal birth after cesarean (VBAC) require less oxygen resuscitation and are less likely to be admitted to neonatal intensive care units (NICU), according to research from Gilbert et al. [23] and Kamath et al. [40]. These infants showed an increase in neonatal infection and a modest rise in transitory tachypnea [23, 40].

The size of the hospital has been found to be a contributing factor to the risk of neonatal death resulting from uterine rupture [29]. Of 107 uterine ruptures in the study by Smith et al. [29], 17 were neonatal deaths of which 13 occurred in hospitals that have <3000 births per annum, 15 in women with no previous vaginal birth, and five associated with the use of prostaglandin as an induction method [29]. In contrast to full uterine ruptures, which resulted in 13.6% more infant deaths than partial uterine ruptures, the partial uterine rupture had no neonatal deaths, according to a study [26]. It is important to highlighted that Keedle et al. [39] emphasized that both qualitative and quantitative studies have shown that having midwifery care can have a positive influence on VBAC rates without an increase in maternal or neonatal morbidity.

2.8 Birth trauma

Many studies on VBAC focus on physical consequences such uterine rupture or surgical trauma with little attention paid to the psychological problems these various birthing methods cause. Birth trauma can result from the emotions that women feel during and after giving birth, not necessarily from the physical mode of delivery. Feelings such as vulnerability, fear, out of control, ignored and abandoned, and anxiety seem to be linked to birth trauma [41, 42]. Traumatic birth has been found to impact on women for many years and can have an impact on lifelong self-esteem and willingness to seek healthcare [43].

Elmir et al. [42] did a review of the literature on birth trauma and found that partner relationships as well as maternal–infant connections may be impacted. Women should have access to counseling and debriefing, according to Elmir et al. who also argue that further study is needed to determine the efficacy of these therapies. Women who give birth via main cesarean may feel any or all of these emotions, and they may or may not have thought about these problems prior to being pregnant again.

In a survey of 59 women who had previously undergone a cesarean section, it was discovered that the previous birth experience was frequently characterized as traumatic and was, on average, scored as scoring 3 out of 10 on a Likert scale, with 1 denoting severe trauma and 10 denoting no trauma [44]. Five themes emerged from the open-ended questions about prior birth experiences, according to the researchers. These themes related to the women's perceived feelings of failure, their sense of control loss, how they were treated by their healthcare providers, their labor and cesarean experiences, and the distress of giving birth apart from their child [44].

The answers after these births were noticeably more positive, with an average rating of 9/10 on the Likert scale. Twenty-nine of the 59 women in this study went on to have a VBAC. The two themes that arose from these encounters were whether or not the women felt in control and how supported they felt [44]. Participants were sourced through a consumer organization called Birthrites, which uses its website to encourage women who want to undergo vaginal birth after cesarean delivery both domestically and overseas. As these women intentionally viewed the website, the authors are aware that this cohort of women is not a representative sample of women who have had cesareans or VBACs. Given the popularity and use of forums and support groups on the internet and in social media, it would be fascinating to replicate this study [44].

The advantages of an after-birth service where women could meet with a midwife consultant on a needs-basis to explore the woman's traumatic birth narrative and to be able to make plans for the next birth were highlighted by a small UK qualitative study that examined women's experiences of a positive birth following a traumatic birth [45]. Five of the study's 14 women (5/14) underwent a cesarean section for their first delivery. Many of these women did not use the service until after their subsequent pregnancies [45]. Women who later had a healthy birth showed sentiments of accomplishment and pride and regarded it as a calming experience; the authors refer to this as a "redemptive birth". This study included two women choosing to have an elective cesarean [45].

3. Summary and conclusions

The eight main themes that concluded in this review were: Women's attitudes and views of VBAC; VBAC education and decision-making programs; previous VBAC; maternal morbidity and mortality in cesarean versus planned VBAC; short inter-pregnancy interval; induction of labor; neonatal morbidity and mortality; and birth trauma.

This review has explored the current issues surrounding VBAC, from the risks of uterine rupture and maternal and neonatal morbidity and mortality to the women's attitudes, views, and experiences. The safety of VBAC has also been explored. Evidence showed that midwife has a positive influence on VBAC rates without an increase in maternal or neonatal morbidity.

Through this literature research, it has been demonstrated that there is a dearth of understanding and knowledge on the factors that might influence a woman's decision to have a VBAC and the views of the midwives who support this choice, so more research is needed to cover this topic deeply. The recommendation drawn from this review is toward increasing the number of VBAC by emphasizing on the midwifery role, continuity of care, personalized care, education program, and conducting more research.

Author details

Eman Alshawish
Faculty of Medicine and Health Sciences, Nursing and Midwifery Department,
An-Najah National University, Nablus, Palestine

*Address all correspondence to: alshawish@najah.edu

References

[1] Cunningham FG, Bangdiwala S, Brown SS. National Institutes of Health Consensus Development Conference Panel. National Institutes of Health Consensus Development conference statement: vaginal birth after cesarean: New insights March 8-10, 2010. Obstetrics & Gynecology. 2010;**115**(6):1279-1295

[2] Clark EA, Silver RM. Long-term maternal morbidity associated with repeat cesarean delivery. American Journal of Obstetrics and Gynecology. 2011;**205**(6 Suppl):S2-S10. DOI: 10.1016/j.ajog.2011.09.028

[3] Guise JM, Eden K, Emeis C, Denman MA, Marshall N, Fu RR, et al. Vaginal birth after cesarean: New insights. Evidence Report/Technology Assessment. 2010;**191**:1-397

[4] Lindquist SAI, Shah N, Overgaard C, Torp-Pedersen C, Glavind K, Larsen T, et al. Association of Previous Cesarean Delivery with Surgical Complications after a hysterectomy later in life. JAMA Surgery. 2017;**152**(12):1148-1155. DOI: 10.1001/jamasurg.2017.2825

[5] McKenna JA, Symon AG. Water VBAC: Exploring a new frontier for women's autonomy. Midwifery. 2014;**30**(1):e20-e25. DOI: 10.1016/j.midw.2013.10.004

[6] Fenwick J, Gamble J, Hauck Y. Believing in birth - choosing VBAC: The childbirth expectations of a self-selected cohort of Australian women. Journal of Clinical Nursing. 2006;**16**:1561-1570

[7] Hadjigeorgiou E, Katsie C, Papadopoulou M, Christofi MD, Christoforou A. Women's experiences of VBAC in Cyprus: A qualitative study. BMC Pregnancy and Childbirth. 2021;**21**(1):766. DOI: 10.1186/s12884-021-04193-7

[8] McGrath P, Phillips E, Vaughan G. Vaginal birth after caesarean risk decision-making: Australian findings on the mothers' perspective. International Journal of Nursing Practice. 2010;**16**:274-281

[9] Meddings F, Phipps FM, Haith-Cooper M, Haigh J. Vaginal birth after caesarean section (VBAC): Exploring women's perceptions. Journal of Clinical Nursing. 2007;**16**(1):160-167. DOI: 10.1111/j.1365-2702.2005.01496.x

[10] Bako B, Geidam AD, Sanusi IM, Mairiga AG, Isa B. Vaginal birth or repeat caesarean section: women's preferred mode of delivery after a primary caesarean section in Maiduguri, Nigeria. International Journal of Medicine and Medical Sciences. 2014;**6**(11):230-235

[11] Dahlen H, Homer C. Motherbirth or childbirth'? A prospective analysis of vaginal birth after caesarean blogs. Midwifery. 2011;**29**(2):167-173. DOI: 10.1016/j.midw.2011.11.007

[12] Emmett C, Shaw ARG, Montgomery AA, Murphy DJ. Women's experience of decision making about mode of delivery after a previous caesarean section: The role of health professionals and information about health risks. BJOG. 2006;**113**:1438-1445

[13] Fraser W, Maunsell E, Hodnett E, Moutquin JM, Childbirth Alternatives Post-Cesarean Study Group. Randomized controlled trial of a prenatal vaginal birth after cesarean section education and support program. American Journal of Obstetrics and Gynecology. 1997;**176**(2):419-425

[14] Frost J, Shaw A, Montgomery A, Murphy DJ. Women's views on the use of decision aids for decision making

about the method of delivery following a previous caesarean section: Qualitative interview study. BJOG: An International Journal of Obstetrics and Gynaecology. 2009;**116**(7):896-905. DOI: 10.1111/j.1471-0528.2009.02120.x

[15] Montgomery A, Emmett CL, Fahey T, Jones C, Ricketts I, Patel RR, et al. Two decision aids for mode of delivery among women with previous caesarean section: Randomised controlled trial. British Medical Journal. 2007;**334**(7607):1305. DOI: 10.1136/bmj.39217.67101955

[16] Wang H-H, Chung U-L, Sung M-S, Wu S-M. Development of a web-based childbirth education program for vaginal birth after C-section (VBAC) mothers. Journal of Nursing Research. 2006;**14**(1):1-7

[17] Nilsson C, Lalor J, Begley C, Carroll M, Gross MM, Grylka-Baeschlin S, et al. Vaginal birth after caesarean: Views of women from countries with low VBAC rates. Women Birth. 2017;**30**:481-490

[18] Nilsson C, van Limbeek E, Vehvilainen-Julkunen K, Lundgren I. Vaginal birth after cesarean: Views of women from countries with high VBAC rates. Qualitative Health Research. 2015;**27**(3):325-340

[19] Mercer BM, Gilbert S, Landon MB, Spong CY, Leveno KJ, Rouse DJ, et al. Labor outcomes with increasing number of prior vaginal births after cesarean delivery. Obstetrics and Gynecology. 2008;**111**(2 Pt 1):285-291. DOI: 10.1097/AOG.0b013e31816102b9

[20] Landon MB, Leindecker S, Spong CY, Hauth JC, Bloom S, Varner MW. The MFMU cesarean registry: Factors affecting the success of trial of labor after previous cesarean delivery. American Journal of Obstetrics and Gynecology. 2005;**193**:1016-1023

[21] Smith GC, White IR, Pell JP, Dobbie R. Predicting caesarean section and uterine rupture among women attempting vaginal birth after prior cesarean section. PLoS Medicine. 2005;**2**:871-878

[22] Crowther CA, Dodd JM, Hiller JE, Haslam RR, Robinson JS, Birth After Caesarean Study Group. Planned vaginal birth or elective repeat caesarean: Patient preference restricted cohort with nested randomised trial. PLoS Medicine. 2012;**9**(3):e1001192. DOI: 10.1371/journal.pmed.1001192

[23] Gilbert SA, Grobman WA, Landon MB, et al. Elective repeat cesarean delivery compared with spontaneous trial of labor after a prior cesarean delivery: A propensity score analysis. American Journal of Obstetrics and Gynecology. 2012;**206**(4):311.e1-311.e9. DOI: 10.1016/j.ajog.2012.02.002

[24] Landon MB, Hauth JC, Leveno KJ, et al. Maternal and perinatal outcomes associated with a trial of labor after prior cesarean delivery. The New England Journal of Medicine. 2004;**351**:2581

[25] Nigam A, Anand R, Jain N. Study of obstetric and fetal outcome of post caesarean pregnancy. International Journal of Reproduction, Contraception Obstetrics and Gynecology. 2015;**4**(1):215

[26] Guiliano M, Closset E, Therby D, LeGoueff F, Deruelle P, Subtil D. Signs, symptoms and complications of complete and partial uterine ruptures during pregnancy and delivery. European Journal of Obstetrics, Gynecology, and Reproductive Biology. 2014;**179**:130-134. DOI: 10.1016/j.ejogrb.2014.05.004

[27] Latendresse G, Murphy PA, Fullerton JT. A description of the management and outcomes of vaginal birth after cesarean birth in the homebirth setting. Journal of Midwifery & Women's Health. 2005;**50**(5):386-391. DOI: 10.1016/j.jmwh.2005.02.012

[28] Stamilio DM, DeFranco E, Paré E, Odibo AO, Peipert JF, Allsworth JE, et al. Short interpregnancy interval: Risk of uterine rupture and complications of vaginal birth after cesarean delivery. Obstetrics and Gynecology. 2007;**110**(5):1075-1082. DOI: 10.1097/01.AOG.0000286759.49895.46

[29] Smith GC, Pell JP, Pasupathy D, Dobbie R. Factors predisposing to perinatal death related to uterine rupture during attempted vaginal birth after caesarean section: Retrospective cohort study. BMJ (Clinical research ed.). 2004;**329**(7462):375. DOI: 10.1136/bmj.38160.634352.55

[30] Buhimschi CS, Buhimschi IA, Patel S, Malinow AM, Weiner CP. Rupture of the uterine scar during term labour: Contractility or biochemistry? BJOG: An International Journal of Obstetrics and Gynaecology. 2005;**112**(1):38-42. DOI: 10.1111/j.1471-0528.2004.00300.x

[31] Fitzpatrick KE, Kurinczuk JJ, Alfirevic Z, Spark P, Brocklehurst P, Knight M. Uterine rupture by intended mode of delivery in the UK: A national case-control study. PLoS Medicine. 2012;**9**(3):e1001184. DOI: 10.1371/journal.pmed.1001184

[32] Stock SJ, Ferguson E, Duffy A, Ford I, Chalmers J, Norman JE. Outcomes of induction of labour in women with previous caesarean delivery: A retrospective cohort study using a population database. PLoS One. 2013;**8**(4):e60404

[33] Palatnik A, Grobman WA. Induction of labor versus expectant management for women with a prior cesarean delivery. American Journal of Obstetrics and Gynecology. 2015;**212**(3):358.e1-358.e3586. DOI: 10.1016/j.ajog.2015.01.026

[34] Wu Y, Kataria Y, Wang Z, et al. Factors associated with successful vaginal birth after a cesarean section: A systematic review and meta-analysis. BMC Pregnancy and Childbirth. 2019;**19**:360. DOI: 10.1186/s12884-019-2517-y

[35] Chen YT, Hsieh Y-C, Shen H, Cheng C-H, Lee K-H, Torng P-L. Vaginal birth after cesarean section: Experience from a regional hospital. Taiwanese Journal of Obstetrics and Gynecology. 2022;**61**(3):422-426. DOI: 10.1016/j.tjog.2022.03.006

[36] Royal College of Obstetricians and Gynaecologists. Birth after Previous Caesarean Birth. Green-top Guideline No. 45. London: RCOG; 2015

[37] Hamdan M, Sidhu K, Sabir N, Omar SZ, Tan PC. Serial membrane sweeping at term in planned vaginal birth after cesarean: A randomized controlled trial. Obstetrics and Gynecology. 2009;**114**(4):745-751. DOI: 10.1097/AOG.0b013e3181b8fa00

[38] Miller ES, Grobman WA. Obstetric outcomes associated with induction of labor after 2 prior cesarean deliveries. American Journal of Obstetrics and Gynecology. 2015;**213**(1):89.e1-89.e5. DOI: 10.1016/j.ajog.2015.02.003

[39] Keedle H, Peters L, Schmied V, et al. Women's experiences of planning a vaginal birth after caesarean in different models of maternity care in Australia. BMC Pregnancy and Childbirth. 2020;**20**:381. DOI: 10.1186/s12884-020-03075-8

[40] Kamath BD, Todd JK, Glazner JE, Lezotte D, Lynch AM. Neonatal outcomes after elective cesarean delivery. Obstetrics and Gynecology. 2009;**113**(6):1231-1238. DOI: 10.1097/AOG.0b013e3181a66d57

[41] Baradaran K. Risk of uterine rupture with vaginal birth after cesarean in twin gestations. Obstetrics and Gynecology International. 2021;**2021**:6693142. DOI: 10.1155/2021/6693142

[42] Elmir R, Schmied V, Wilkes L, Jackson D. Women's perceptions and experiences of a traumatic birth: A meta-ethnography. Journal of Advanced Nursing. 2010;**66**(10):2142-2153. DOI: 10.1111/j.1365-2648.2010.05391.x

[43] Forssen AS. Lifelong significance of disempowering experiences in prenatal and maternity care: Interviews with elderly Swedish women. Qualitative Health Research. 2012;**22**(11):1535-1546. DOI: 10.1177/1049732312449212

[44] Fenwick J, Gamble J, Mawson J. Women's experiences of Caesarean section and vaginal birth after Caesarian: A Birthrites initiative. International Journal of Nursing Practice. 2003;**9**(1):10-17

[45] Thomson G, Downe S. Changing the future to change the past: Women's experience of a positive birth following a traumatic birth experience. Journal of Reproductive and Infant Psychology. 2010;**28**(1):102-112

Section 4

Robotic Surgery

Chapter 6

Robotically Assisted Hysterectomy

Petre Bratila, Anca Manta, Alexandra Paun and Elvira Bratila

Abstract

Starting from the first robotic hysterectomy, currently, this method is widely accepted all over the world as an alternative to open or laparoscopic surgery due to the technical advantages it offers. We are currently using the DaVinci Xi platform, whose components, instruments, and accessories are described. This chapter aims to present all surgical steps of a robotically assisted hysterectomy, starting with patient positioning, uterine manipulator insertion, port insertion, pneumoperitoneum performing, and the operative technique of the total robotic hysterectomy: connective vascular disconnection, colpotomy, uterus retrieval, and colporrhaphy. A special mention belongs to radical robotic hysterectomy with sentinel node detection and pelvic lymphadenectomy. The chapter ends with a brief description of the perioperative complications.

Keywords: robotics, hysterectomy, surgical technique, minimally-invasive, artificial intelligence, robotically assisted hysterectomy, Da Vinci Xi platform, surgical steps

1. Introduction

The idea of using robotic systems in surgery was proposed as early as 1967; it took more than 30 years of study and thorough research to complete the first fully multifunctional surgical robot. The first robotic System used was ROBODOC, used in orthopedic surgery for hip prosthesis; it was developed and used by Hap Paul and William Bargar in late 1980 [1–3]. Subsequently, systems were created and used in urology, prostate surgery, neurosurgery, otorhinolaryngology, gynecology, and cardiovascular surgery [4].

The United States Department of Defense developed the concept of robotic surgery to provide fast, high-precision surgical assistance directly on the battlefield. The prototype built contained two separate units: the surgeon's working unit and a remote-controlled surgical unit [5]. The System consisted of two video cameras that sent images from the operating field to a remote console. The surgeon could safely steer the robot's arms, thus accessing surgical instruments. This prototype has undergone several changes and improvements over time [6].

There are currently three types of robotic surgical systems: the AESOP, the Da Vinci System, and the ZEUS System. Currently, an essential multifunctional robotic surgery system approved by the FDA is the Da Vinci type from intuitive surgical Inc., which is used worldwide. The Da Vinci System comprises the surgeon's console, the video system, and the patient's cart, containing three or four robotic arms. The surgeon at the work console remotely directs the instruments attached to the robot arms [7].

In 1997, the first Da Vinci prototype was tested in humans, demonstrating the effectiveness of multiple joint instruments in abdominal and cardiovascular surgery. The FDA approved using this System in surgical practice in 2000 [8]. Since 2005, the Da Vinci System has been approved in the United States for use in gynecological procedures, both benign and malignant. The most highly-performed major surgical procedure in gynecology is a hysterectomy [9].

The first simple robotic hysterectomy was performed in 2002, and the first radical robotic hysterectomy was completed four years later, in 2006 [10]. The robotic hysterectomy is widely accepted as an alternative to open or laparoscopic surgery due to the technical advantages of robotic surgery, including 3-dimensional viewing, more precise control of instruments, and further articulation of tools, which enable surgeries to perform complex procedures more carefully. Minimally invasive robotic surgery is used today for up to 30% of benign and up to 65% of oncology cases in gynecologic surgery [11].

1.1 The robot: DaVinci Xi last generation

The DaVinci Xi platform is the 4th generation of the Da Vinci System.

The System has four components: surgeon console, patient cart, vision cart, and electrosurgery unit.

1.1.1 The Surgeon Console

The Surgeon Console provides an ergonomic design for the surgeon's comfort during surgery. It has a 3D Viewer, which enhances the vision of anatomy, and hand controls, which have intuitive motion translated into precise, delicate, tremor-filtered movements at instrument tips (**Figure 1**).

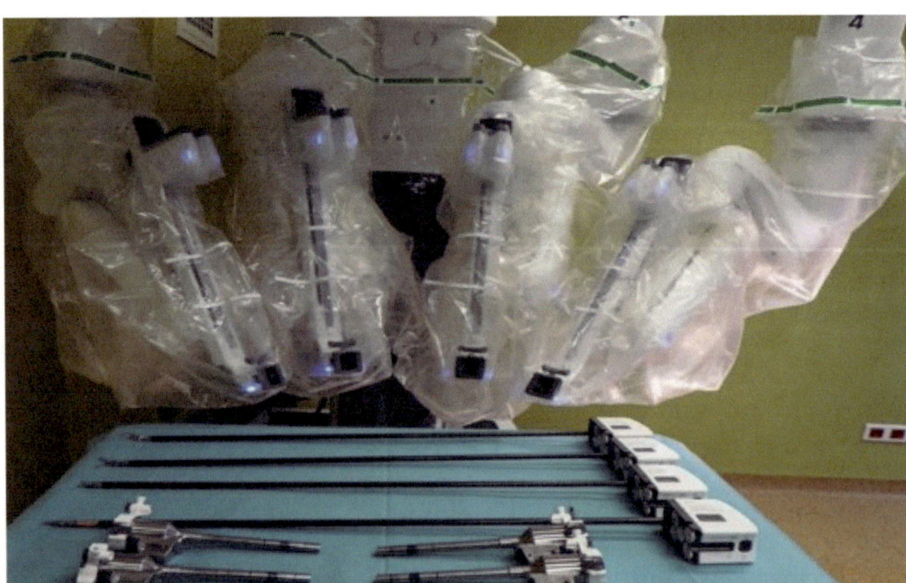

Figure 1.
A patient cart, trocars, and instruments.

DOI: http://dx.doi.org/10.5772/intechopen.112144

1.1.2 The Patient Cart

This presents an adjustable support structure named boom which offers flexibility in positioning his arms over the surgical table. It has universal arms which allow the assignment and re-configuration of endoscope and instruments to desired ports during a surgical procedure.

The Helm touchpad allows non-sterile OR Staff to select the Patient Cart setting and adjust boon height or position for the best efficiency.

1.1.3 The Vision Cart

It is composed of a touchscreen monitor, an ERBE VIO dV generator, and an endoscope controller. The Endoscope controller provides a high-intensity light source to illuminate the surgical site and houses electronics that promote efficient endoscope setup.

The touchscreen monitor provides a high-quality view of the surgical image and allows non-sterile OR Staff to adjust vision settings and troubleshoot faults.

1.1.4 The electrosurgical unit

An ERBE VIO dV generator is integrated with the System; this electrosurgical unit (ESU) indicates the location of installed energy instruments and displays the energy effect setting at the surgeon console, increasing surgeon autonomy.

1.2 Instruments and accessories

1.2.1 The access instruments

- 8 mm cannulas, 5–8 mm cannula seals, 8 mm blunt obturator, 8 mm bladeless obturator and an 8 mm 0° or 30° endoscope

The endoscope allows magnified 3D High-Definition vision and provides a consistently clear view of the surgical field. The surgeon can adjust up or down 30° cameras according to the necessities. The camera can change vision in infrared.

1.2.2 Surgical instruments

- Monopolar curved scissors are protected by a neutral tip cover.

- Fenestrated bipolar forceps are used for grasping, retraction, dissection, and bipolar coagulation of the tissue.

- Maryland bipolar forceps are used for the same action as fenestrated bipolar forceps,

- Non-energy grasper (Cadiere grasper)

- Needle drivers
- Prograsp forceps

Special devices can be adapted to the arms of the robot as:

- *Synchro Seal* enables to seal and cut of vessels up to 5 mm in diameter and tissue bundles that fit in the jaws. The average sealing time is less than 2 s.
- *Vessel Sealer Extend* securely seals and cut vessels up to 7 mm in diameter or tissue bundles that fit in the jaws. The sealing time is less than 3 s. It presents four functions: grasp, dissect, seal, and cut.
- *Ultracision* seal and cut tissues using ultrasounds, best used for robotic myomectomy (**Figures 2–10**).

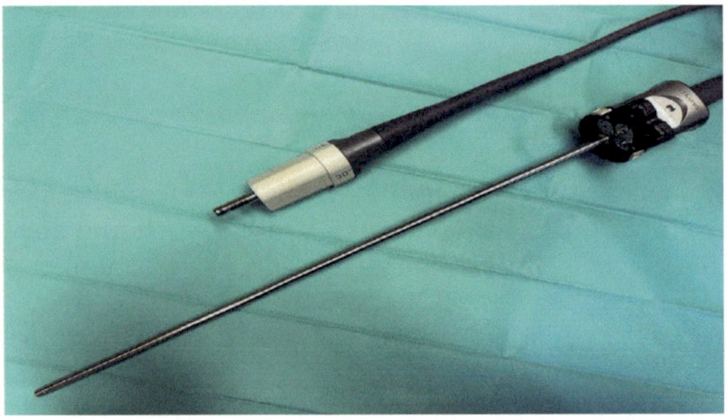

Figure 2.
3D camera.

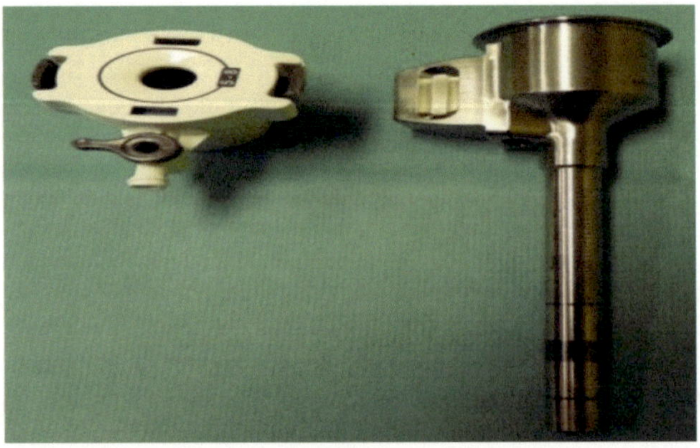

Figure 3.
Canula and canula seals.

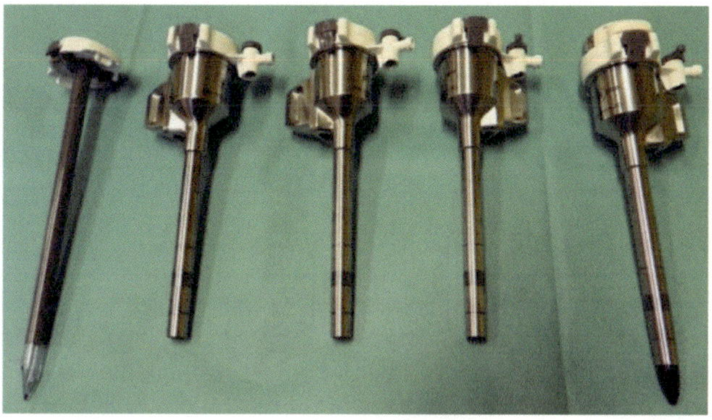

Figure 4.
Cannulas with a bladeless and blunt obturator.

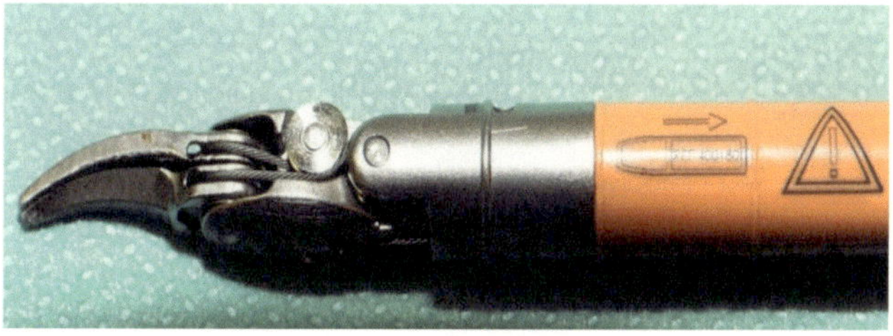

Figure 5.
Monopolar curved scissors.

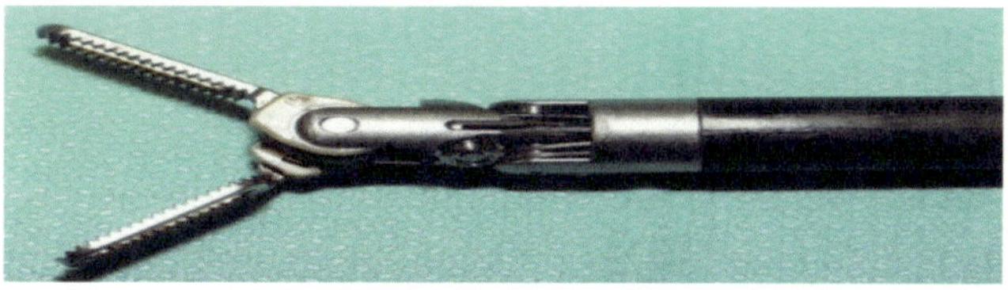

Figure 6.
Bipolar fenestrated forceps.

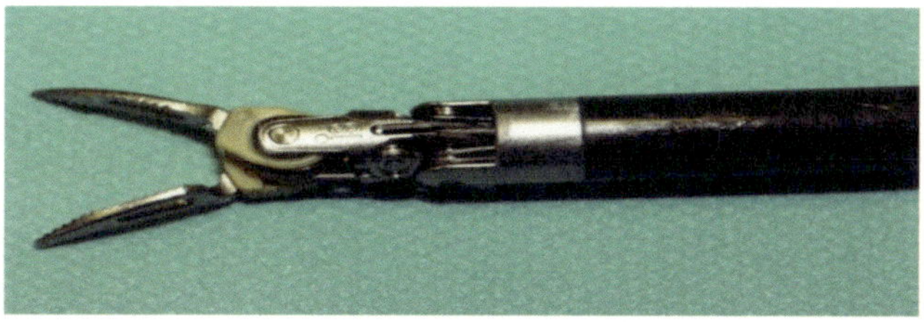

Figure 7.
Maryland bipolar forceps.

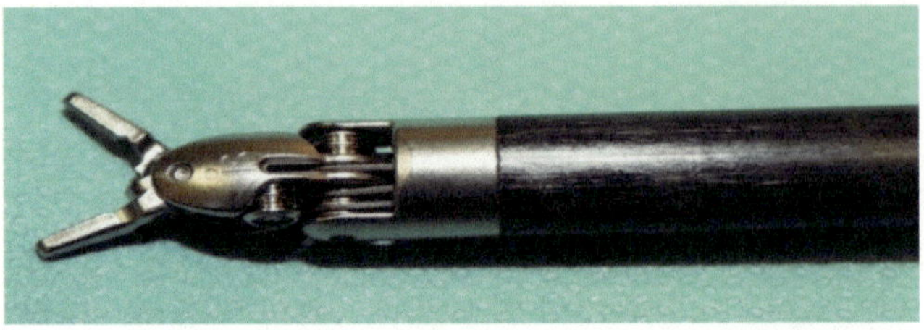

Figure 8.
Large needle driver.

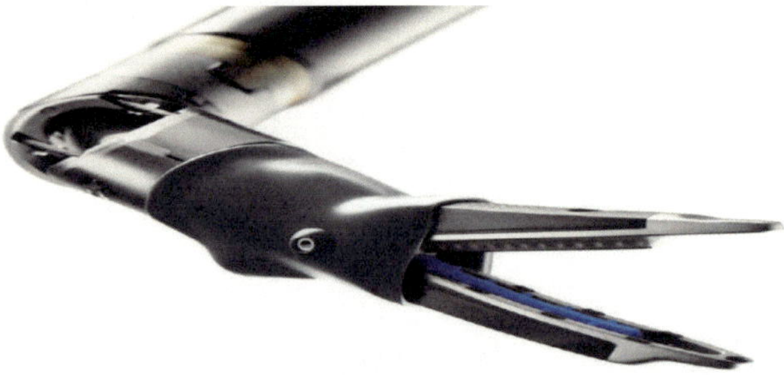

Figure 9.
SynchroSeal @Intuitive Corporation Sunnyvale, CA, USA (Sofmedica, Romania).

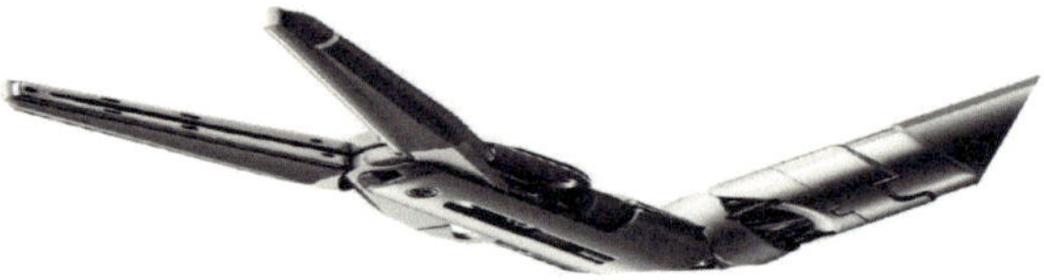

Figure 10.
Vessel Sealer Extend @Intuitive Corporation Sunnyvale, CA, USA (Sofmedica, Romania).

2. Operation theater setup and operative access

2.1 Patient positioning and the uterine manipulator insertion

The uterine manipulator allows to move the uterus up and down or in a lateral position. To facilitate the insertion of a uterine manipulator, the patient must be placed in a lithotomy position with legs in stirrups and spread apart in slight ventral flexion. The buttocks must be placed slightly over the edge of the operating table, a position that allows movements of the uterine manipulator.

A bladder catheter is inserted before the uterine manipulator placement.

The patient arms must be placed along the body to avoid injury to the brachial plexus.

We use the Koh manipulator with three different cups according to the dimensions of the cervix and vagina. For robotic surgery, we need a prominent Trendelenburg position (25–30°). The shoulder braces are mandatory to avoid slipping.

2.2 Abdominal access. First port insertion. Pneumoperitoneum

In most cases, the access for the vision port is done transumbilical. The umbilical area is the thinnest abdominal wall area, where aponeurosis detaches difficult from the peritoneum.

We anchor the umbilicus with two forceps, and a small incision of the skin is made to allow the insertion of the Veress needle. The correct positioning of the Veress needle inside the peritoneum is checked using known tests: suction, drop, or pressure tests. For abdominal placement of the vision port, the surgical table must be placed in a neutral position to avoid the risk of vascular injury of great vessels.

The pneumoperitoneum, for gynecological surgeries, is done to a pressure of 12–15 mmHg. To allow the insertion of an 8 mm trochar, the umbilical incision will be extended. The trochar is inserted perpendicular to the abdominal wall with the shutter mounted. When removed the shutter, a gas jet under pressure is heard, a sign that the instrument is correctly placed. Connect the cannula tap to the CO2 insufflation system and insert the camera [11, 12].

Other methods of making pneumoperitoneum, the Henson trochar approach, the visiport trochar, or the Veress optical needle, are rarely used [12].

2.3 Ancillary trochars placement

The working trochars are inserted under visual control. The incision in the skin will be about 8 mm to allow the tight insertion of the trocar. We use, for gynecological surgery, 3 or 4 Da Vinci trochars and one assistant's trochar placed in line. In the case of a simple robotic hysterectomy, we put four trochars in the umbilical cord. The distance between the trochars should be about 8–10 cm to avoid crossing the instruments during surgery. For fragile patients, the holes can be placed at distances of up to 4 cm without exceeding this value. The Da Vinci system trochars, marked with three black lines, are inserted so that the midline is placed at the level of the peritoneum.

The assistant surgeon uses a 12 mm trochar to couple the Air Seal system. It is placed on the right or left side, either on the umbilical line or triangular and cranial, between the optical and Da Vinci 2 or 3 ports.

The distance between the assistant and Da Vinci ports must exceed 7 cm.

Place the patient in the Trendelenburg position at 25‾30°. In the case of the adjoining syndrome, under visual control, adhesiolysis is performed. Remove the small intestine and epiploon from the visual field with an atraumatic pen. Place the surgical table in the lowest position possible. Dock arm 2 of the Da Vinci System at the endoscopic port. Insert the 8 mm 30 degrees endoscope and target the pubic symphysis. Arms 2 and 3 are docked.

The work tools are inserted as follows: on arm 2, the bipolar or vessel sealer extends is mounted, and on arm three is mounted monopolar curved scissors. Arm 4 will remain stowed (**Figure 11**).

3. The robotic hysterectomy

Hysterectomy is one of the most common non-pregnancy-related gynecological surgeries. There are three main types of hysterectomy [13]: *Total hysterectomy*, *Supracervical* hysterectomy, and *Radical hysterectomy*. The uni- or bilateral adnexectomy or salpingectomy can be associated with any type of hysterectomy.

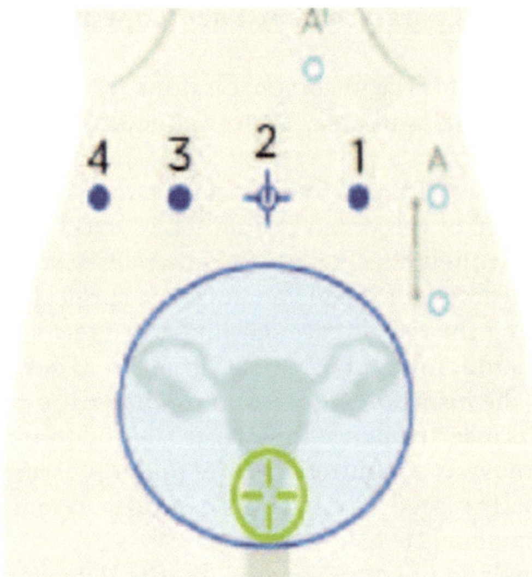

Figure 11.
Ancilliary trochars placement for Xi platform.

- *Total robotic hysterectomy* can be indicated for benign disease of the uterus or the early stages of endometrial cancer.

The specific indications for robotic assistance are:

- Morbid obesity
- Big uterus
- Previous complicated surgeries
- Deep infiltrating endometriosis
- Patient preference

For benign and malignant conditions robotic hysterectomy is equivalent to a type A hysterectomy in the Querleu Morrow classification. It represents an extra fascial hysterectomy in which all the uterine pedicles are resected as close to the uterus as possible. The area of the cut of the vagina is <10 mm. Ureterolysis is not necessary, but ureters must only be identified. The main advantage of this type of hysterectomy consists of the possibilities of uterus extraction in a natural way, through the vagina.

- *Supracervical hysterectomy*- involves the removal only of the uterine body. The cervix is preserved. The main indication for supracervical hysterectomy is the express desire of the patient to keep the cervix for benign uterine conditions such as dysfunctional bleeding resistant to treatment, uterine leiomyomatosis, and uterine adenomyosis. Supravaginal hysterectomy can be performed in cases when technically the cervix cannot be extracted. After a supravaginal hysterectomy, the uterine body cannot be extracted vaginally. The alternatives are in-bag morcellation and morcellation by mini-laparotomy.

- *Radical hysterectomy* remains the standard surgical treatment for the different early types of cervical cancer and endometrial cancer. If for early cervical cancer, the lymphadenectomy is mandatory for endometrial cancer stage, I or II it must respect the molecular classification and degree of risk. The real radical hysterectomy is represented by Types B and C from Querleu Morrow's classification.

Current guidelines from NCCN and ESGO indicated that both open surgery and minimally invasive surgery performed by conventional (laparoscopy) or robotic techniques are acceptable approaches to radical hysterectomy with pelvic lymphadenectomy in patients with early-stage cervical cancer and endometrial cancer [14–17]. The retrospective study showed that robot-assisted radical hysterectomy was associated with better perioperative outcomes than the open approach, and the recurrence rates and survival rates do not differ significantly between these two ways of performing radical hysterectomies [14, 17].

3.1 Total robotic hysterectomy-operative technique

The robotic hysterectomy starts with an abdominal cavity inspection. Once the pneumoperitoneum was created, we checked the trochar's placement and the presence of possible intestinal or vascular trochar insertion injuries.

All four quadrants of the abdominal cavity must be inspected, including the liver and diaphragm.

The whole pelvis will be exposed after we mobilize the small bowel and sigmoid and perform adhesiolysis if it is necessary. Uterine and adnexa inspection aim to check the adequate uterine manipulator insertion and anatomy of the adnexa, the position of ureters, and the vascular axes of the pelvis.

The technique of total hysterectomy requires *disconnecting of the uterus* and cervix from vascular and connective elements of the supporting System, *section of the vagina*, *extraction* of the uterus, and *closing of* the vaginal cuff.

3.2 Connective vascular disconnection

The uterus is kept in anatomical position at three levels of connective vascular pedicles: *the superior pedicle* consisting of round ligaments and utero-adnexal or infundibulopelvic ligaments, the *medium vascular pedicle* represented by leading uterine vessels and the *inferior pedicle* consisting of cervicovaginal vessels. Only the superior pedicle is intraperitoneal, the medium and inferior being between the two folds of large ligaments. The disconnection will be done by both sides of the uterus.

3.2.1 Superior pedicle disconnection

- Starts with coagulation and sectioning of *the round ligament* at the level of the avascular triangle of the broad ligament. The triangle is limited by adnexal vessels medially, extern iliac vessels laterally, and round ligament caudally (**Figure 12**).

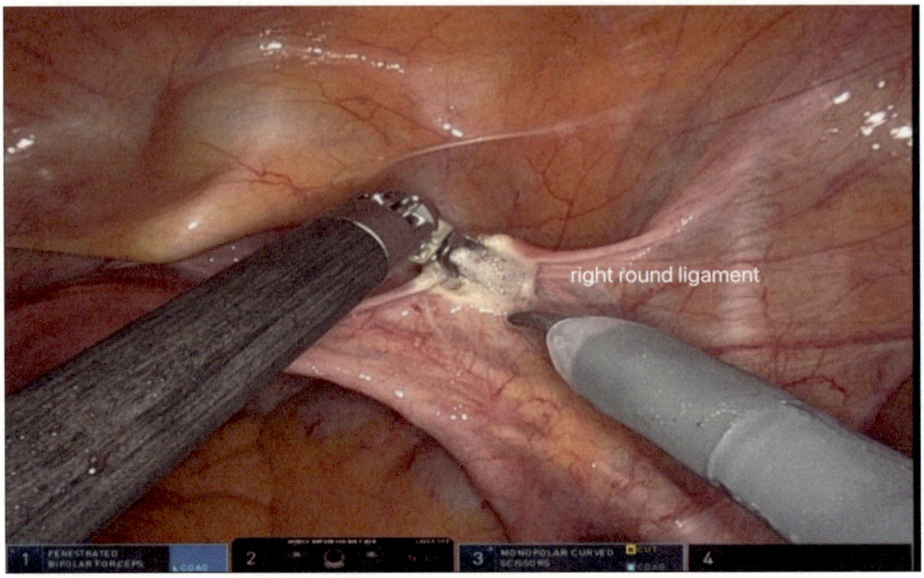

Figure 12.
Coagulation and section of the right round ligament.

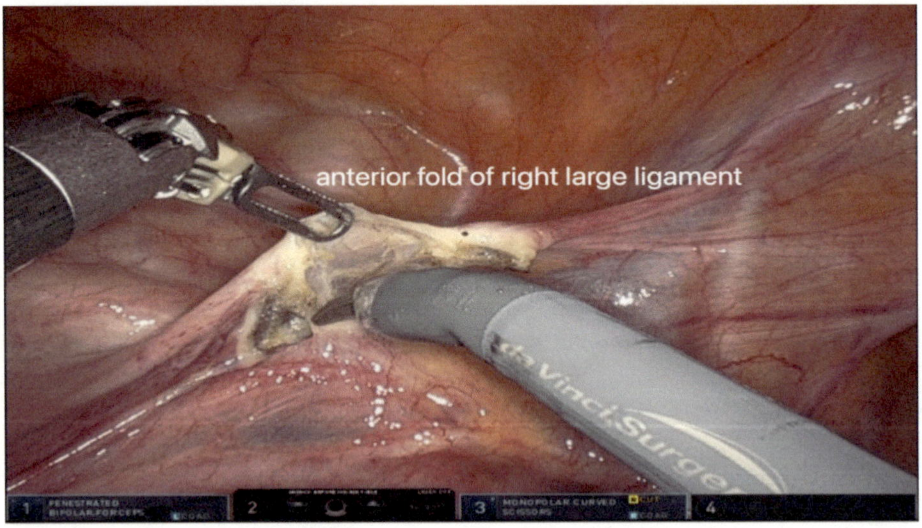

Figure 13.
Sectioning of the anterior fold of broad ligament.

- Division of *anterior and posterior fold of the broad ligament* and entrance in the retroperitoneal space. Sectioning of the anterior fold of the broad ligament, by dissection and coagulation towards the medial vesical line (**Figure 13**).

- Coagulation and section of *utero-ovarian or infundibulopelvic ligaments* (left and right). We recommend at first performing fenestration of the broad ligament at

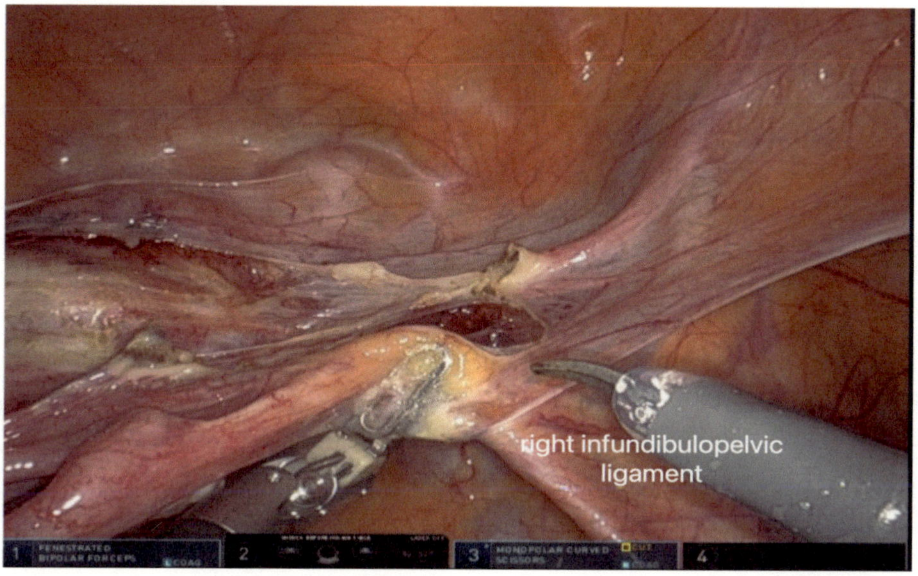

Figure 14.
Coagulating and division of the infundibulopelvic ligament.

the level of the gray triangle. This maneuver allows to check the position of the ureter in the dissection area (**Figure 14**).

- *Utero-ovarian pedicle* disconnection will be done by separate coagulation and sectioning of the fallopian tube and utero-ovarian ligament. An important vascular anastomosis between the two elements links the fundal uterine artery and veins to the tubo-ovarian arcade. The level of the section must be in the gray triangle away from uterine insertion.

- *Infundibulopelvic disconnection* is an important step concerning the risk of ureteral injury. Before coagulating the ligament, it must be skeletonized by a section of the peritoneum in the direction of external iliac vessels. The ureter is just under the pedicle. The coagulation will be done step by step in the direction of the fenestrated large ligament.

3.2.2 Dissection of the vesicouterine space

Sectioning the anterior fold of the broad ligament allows for dissecting the vesicouterine space. The junction of the peritoneum between the bladder and uterus looks like a white line. The incision of the peritoneum must be performed caudal to this line (**Figures 15** and **16**).

In the case of previous cesarean sections, this limit is hard to see, and entering into the cervico-vesical space is difficult. Dissection will be made step by step searching the contact with the manipulator cup. After entering the vesico-cervico-vaginal space the limit between the bladder and vagina is cervicovaginal fascia visible as a white connective structure. The assistant grasps the bladder at the midline by anterior and superior traction and dissection is carried out in the midline. Laterally the bladder pillars must be coagulated and cut bilaterally.

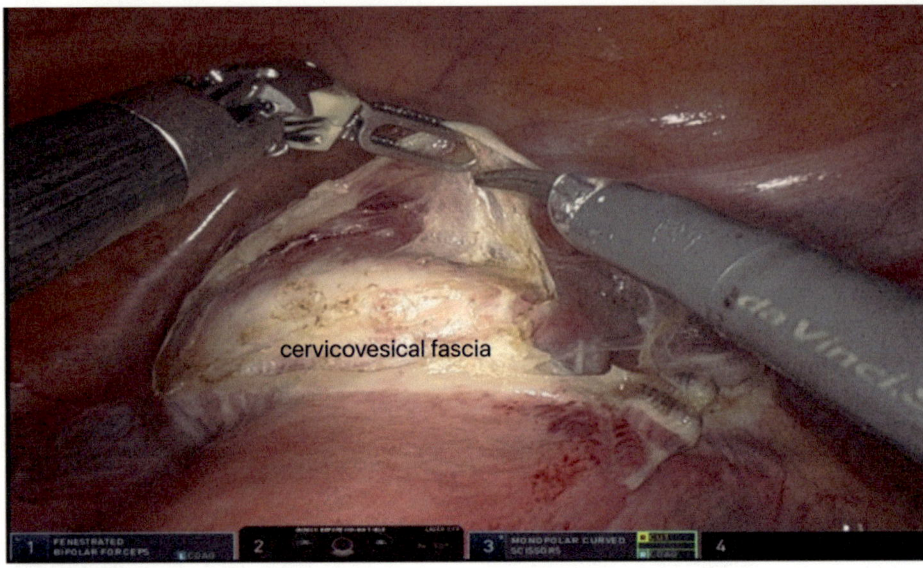

Figure 15.
Dissection of vesicouterine space.

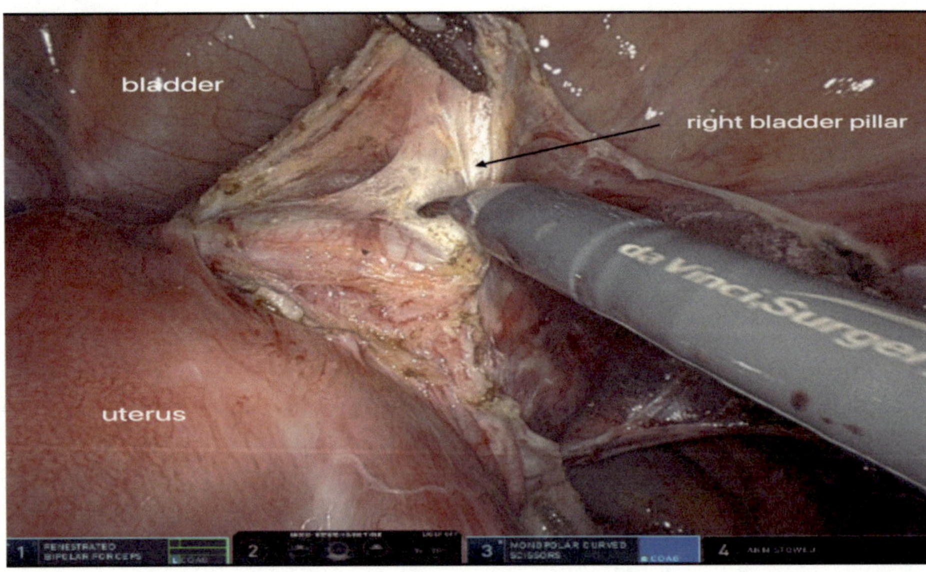

Figure 16.
Right bladder pillar.

3.2.3 Disconnection of the leading vascular pedicle

The first step to disconnect the leading vascular pedicle is to skeletonize the uterine vascular axes. It should be remembered that the division of the uterine artery is done at the level of the uterine isthmus. Here the main trunk is divided into an ascending and a descending branch. In this operative step, only the ascendant branch of the uterine artery is coagulated and sectioned.

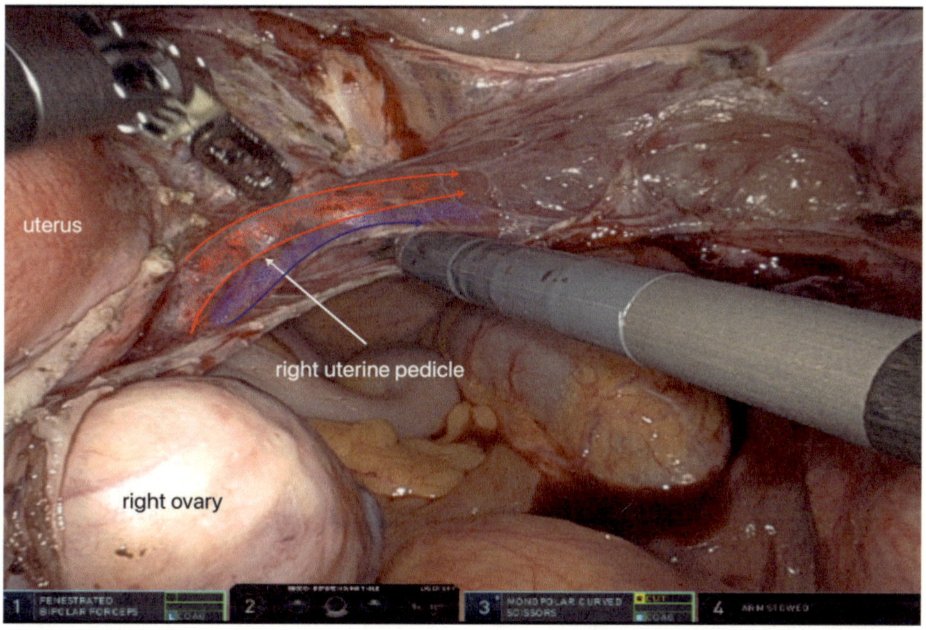

Figure 17.
Scheletonize the right uterine pedicle artery and vein.

To highlight the uterine vascular axis the posterior broad ligament peritoneum must be sectioned towards the uterosacral ligaments. In the vascular pedicle, the artery is located before the veins and the bleeding is easy to control. If the artery has a diameter of more than 5 mm a haemoclip is useful to control arterial bleeding (**Figure 17**).

3.2.4 Disconnecting the inferior connective vascular pedicle

The inferior connective vascular pedicle contains *a vascular part* represented by a descending branch of the uterine artery, cervicovaginal vessels, vaginal artery and veins, and the *fibrous supporting System* of the uterus that contains the cardinal uterosacral complex (CUSC).

For the ascendant branch of the uterine artery hemostasis is done with the bipolar clamp placed perpendicular to the axis of the uterus. For cervicovaginal vessels, coagulation and sectioning of are done parallel to the uterine axis. Usually, we do not coagulate and section the uterosacral ligaments separately. In some cases, with a big uterus, the coagulation and section of the uterosacral ligaments can help mobilize the uterus and facilitate the colpotomy (**Figure 18**).

3.3 Colpotomy

The colpotomy is an important step of robotic hysterectomy because if done correctly it prevents several complications to neighboring organs: ureteral, bladder, and rectum. To prevent these complications some rules must be followed:

- Do not dissect too much lower the inferior pedicle. The ureter is inside the bladder pillar.

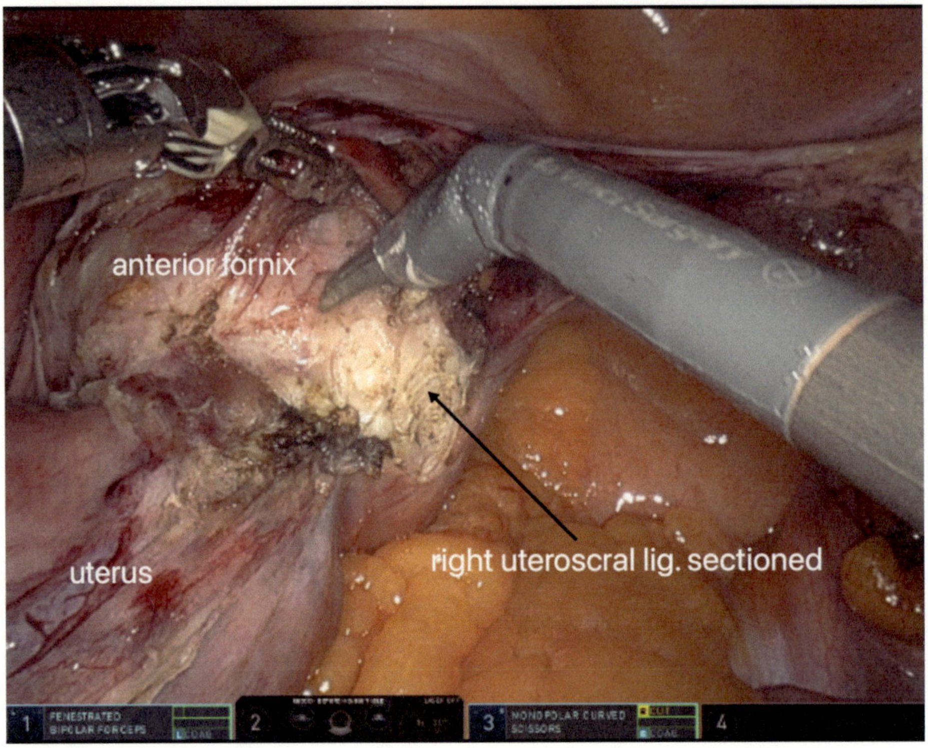

Figure 18.
Inferior pedicle. Cervicovaginal vessels are coagulated and sectioned. Right uterosacral ligament exposed and divided.

- If the CUSC is strong start the colpotomy posteriorly sectioning it.
- Completely frees the vaginal fornices.
- Be careful with adhesions to the torus of the uterus.
- Do not use excessive bipolar current to control hemostasis.
- Circumferential colpotomy starting at the lateral sides performed by monopolar scissors (**Figure 19**).

3.4 Extraction (uterus retrieval)

In most cases with big uteri, the time-consuming retrieval exceeds the time for uterus disconnection. In cases of a uterus weighing under 280gr vaginal retrieval is not a problem.

For the big uteri we can use other alternatives:

- Transvaginal morcelation
- In bag morcelation

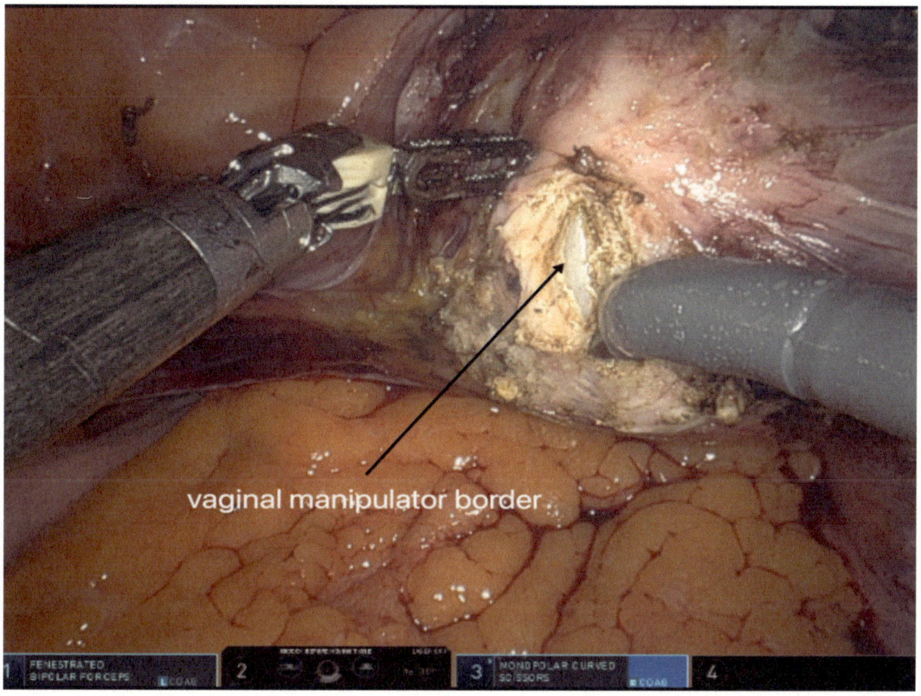

Figure 19.
Colpotomy starts from the lateral side of the vaginal cuff.

- Power morcelation
- Cutting morcelation (Chardoney)
- Minilaparotomy and morcelation

Transvaginal morcellation is the leading method for uterus extraction. For the surgeon trained in vaginal surgery extraction of a uterus weighing 500–1000 gr is not a problem. To extract the uterus transvaginally, we use some techniques:

- Hemisection (bivalve)
- Intramiometrial corring (Lash technique)
- Wedge morcellation
- A combination of these techniques

After colpotomy, the entire uterus remains free into the pelvis if the manipulator is extracted. The vaginal assistant grasps the cervix with a tenaculum pulling it into the vaginal canal.

Usually, we start transvaginal morcellation bilvalving of the uterus beginning from the external cervical orifice. This maneuver allows access to the lateral sides of the uterine body allowing to start the intramiometrial corring. The uterine body tissue is cut circularly with a knife or scissors forming a cylinder of tissue to reduce the volume of the uterus. If necessary, tissue fragments can be cut for uterine reduction. Finally, the whole uterus will be extracted vaginally.

3.5 Colporraphy

Closing the vagina is the final step of hysterectomy. We close the vagina by continuous uninterrupted sutures in one layer, including enough width of the vaginal mucosa, fascia, and uterosacral ligaments to strengthen pelvic support. We use resorbable suture (Vycril no. 1) or barbed suture No.00 (**Figure 20**).

3.6 Final step

Hemostasis and final inspection and pelvis irrigation and aspiration. We check vascular pedicles, vaginal vaults, ureters, and bladder. We check the presence of unapparent injuries in surrounding structures. We lower intra-abdominal pressure to 9 mmHg to see the hemostasis efficiency. We practice routine pelvic drainage for 24 h to prevent postoperative bleeding.

Undocking the platform is the next step. The trochars are removed under direct vision and we check parietal hemostasis. The pneumoperitoneum is exusuflated.

We close the fascia of the umbilical and assistant port. The skin incisions are closed with a subcuticular suture.

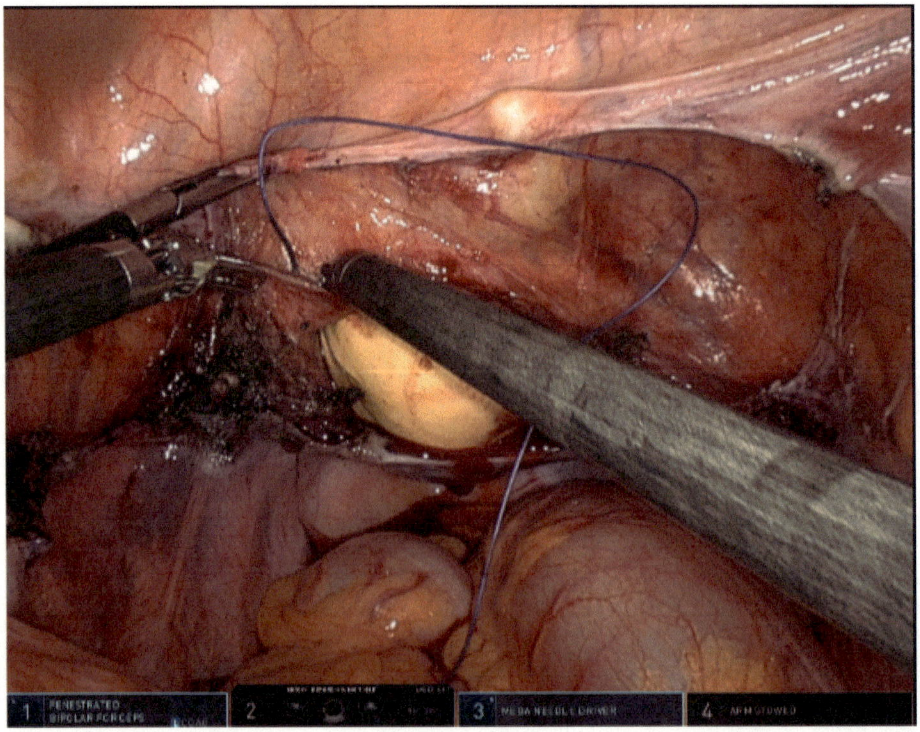

Figure 20.
Closing the vagina in one layer with running uninterrupted suture.

3.6.1 Radical robotic hysterectomy

Radical hysterectomy with pelvic lymphadenectomy with or without adnexectomy remains the standard recommended surgical treatment for the different types of gynecological cancer. Depending on the type of cancer (cervical, endometrial, or ovarian), one of the types of radical hysterectomy from the Querleu classification and pelvic lymphadenectomy is performed [13, 14, 18].

Radical robotic hysterectomy is indicated for the early stages of cervical and endometrial cancer. In most cases, the procedure can be associated with pelvic or paraortic lymphadenectomy. If for cervical invasive cancer, the lymphadenectomy is mandatory for endometrial cancer lymphadenectomy aims at surgical staging.

The first part of the procedure is like all types of hysterectomies. It involves the disconnection of the superior connective vascular pedicle and the dissection of the bladder from the cervix and vagina [19]. For all the procedures the vascular pedicle sealing is performed using electrosurgical instruments: bipolar clamp, ultrasound clamp, Vessel Sealer Extend, or SynchroSeal.

Surgical staging with pelvic lymphadenectomy with or without para-aortic lymphadenectomy defines recurrence risk and determines the clinician's decision to give patients adjuvant treatment (radiation or chemotherapy) [15]. Systematic surgical staging significantly reduces the necessity of external radiation, avoiding the complications of complete pelvic lymphadenectomy [20–23].

The concept of the sentinel lymph node (SLN) has been proposed as a less invasive solution for nodal assessment. The state of the sentinel node ganglion reflects the status of the entire nodal basin of pelvic lymph nodes [24–26] (**Figure 21**).

The leading step of radical hysterectomy is the dissection of parametria. The extension of parametrial resection is decided according to the clinical stage of the tumor. For stage IB of the cervix and stage II for endometrial cancer is recommended parametrial resection C2 and pelvic lymphadenectomy. For stage I endometrial cancer SLN detection and B2 are recommended (**Figures 22** and **23**).

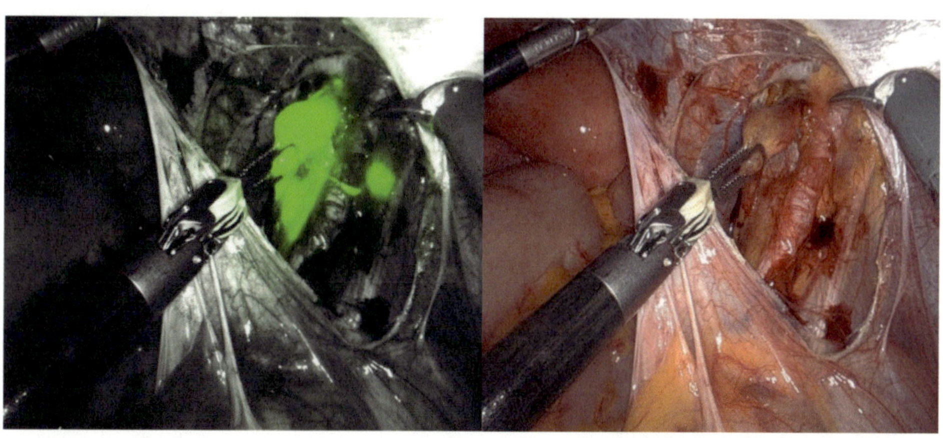

Figure 21.
SLN detection in obturator right fossa after 20 min after ICG intrastromal cervical injection.

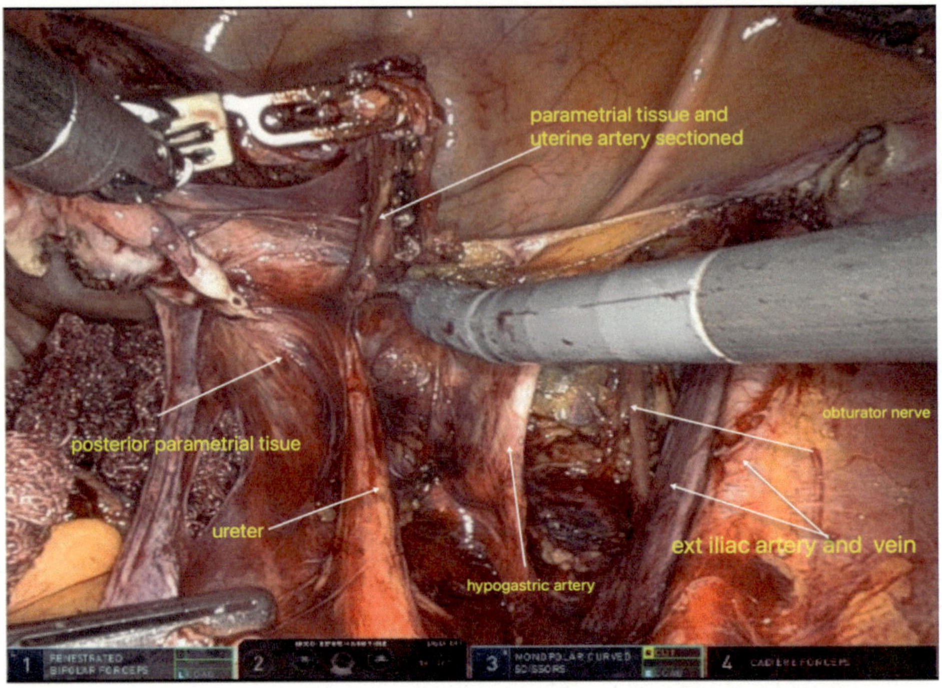

Figure 22.
Right side parametrectomy. The parametrial tissue is lifting to allow unroofing of the ureter.

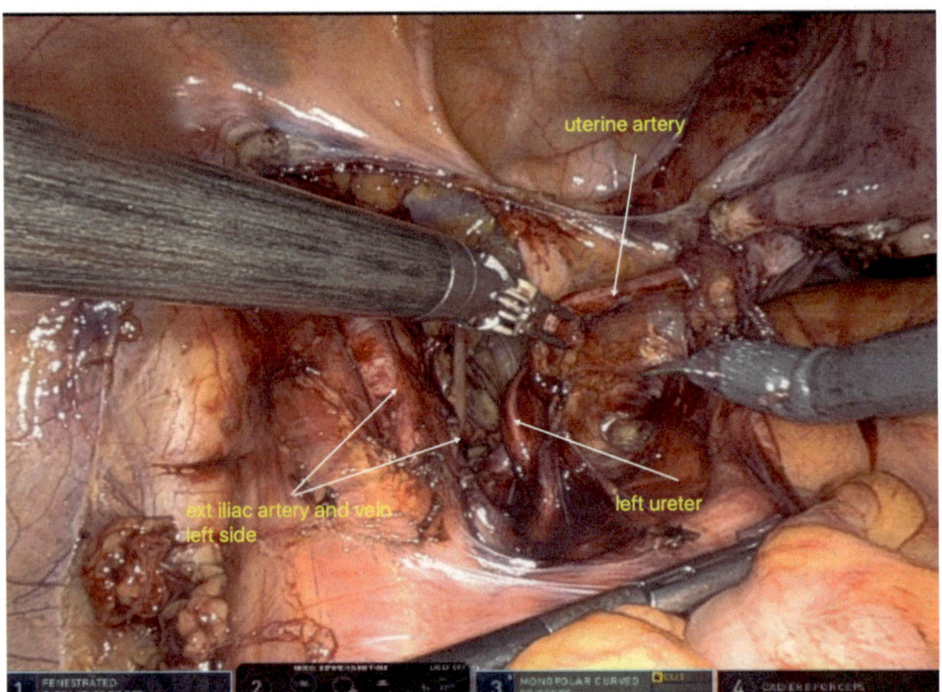

Figure 23.
Left side parametrectomy. Opening the Lazko space. The uterine artery can be seen crossing the left ureter.

4. Perioperative complications of robotic hysterectomy

Possible postoperative complications include fever, respiratory failure and pneumonia, postoperative ileus, sepsis, transfusion need, urine retention, and parietal complications [27–31].

Fever is the most common secondary complication of hysterectomy. The most common causes are urinary or respiratory tract infections. Most of the time, however, the etiology of fever is unclear; in patients with robotic interventions, it is not associated with increased sepsis, wound infections, or pneumonia. One possible explanation would be that it appears secondary to the atelectasis related to the increased duration of the Trendelenburg position [32].

The leading risk factor for *respiratory complications*, is the generally longer operating times in steep Trendelenburg position in robotic-operated patients [33].

The factors related to *urinary retention* in robotic hysterectomy patients remain unknown [28]. The solution is maintaining an indwelling urinary catheter for at least one day after a hysterectomy, especially in elderly patients.

Intraoperative complications are classified into hemorrhagic, digestive, and urinary tract complications. The occurrence of any of these complications can cause laparoscopic or laparotomic conversion. Most complications occur when inserting the first trocar. The most severe complication is bleeding from damage to large vessels [34, 35].

Intraoperative *hemorrhagic complications* in robotic interventions are rare, with a reduced need for transfusions compared to other types of hysterectomies [27].

Bladder injuries can occur during bladder-uterine dissection, being favored by a history of cesarean section. In particular, this type of injury is more common in radical interventions than in standard total hysterectomies because radical hysterectomy involves extensive dissection of periureteral tissue, unroofing of the ureteral tunnel, and the mobilization of the blender, It is essential to recognize them intraoperative. The incidence of bladder injuries during radical hysterectomy is between 0.4 and 3.7%.

Ureteral lesions depend on the complexity of the intervention, with a variable incidence between 0.08 and 4.2%. Most commonly, they occur through thermal injury or radical hysterectomy. The appearance of uterovaginal fistulas follows their non-recognition. The incidence of vesicovaginal and uterovaginal fistulas is between 0.9 and 2.0% [35–37].

Author details

Petre Bratila[1*], Anca Manta[1], Alexandra Paun[1] and Elvira Bratila[2]

1 Gynecology Department, Minimally Invasive Surgery Euroclinic Hospital "Regina Maria", Bucharest, Romania

2 Medicine and Pharmacy University "Carol Davila", Bucharest, Romania

*Address all correspondence to: pbratila49@yahoo.com

References

[1] Corliss WR, Johnson EG. Teleoperators and Human Augmentation. An AEC-NASA Technology Survey. Washington, DC: Office of Technology Utilization, National Aeronautics, and Space Administration; 1967

[2] Paul HA, Bargar WL, Mittlestadt B, et al. Development of a surgical robot for cementless total hip arthroplasty. Clinical Orthopaedics and Related Research. 1992;**285**:57-66

[3] Davies BL, Ng W, Hibberd RD. Prostatic resection: An example of safe robotic surgery. Robotica. 1993;**11**:561-566

[4] Harris S, Arambula-Cosio F, Mei Q, et al. The Probot—An active robot for prostate resection. Proceedings of the Institution of Mechanical Engineers, Part H: The New England Journal of Medicine. 1997;**211**:317-325

[5] Zajtchuk R, Grande C. Part IV. Surgical Combat Casualty Care: Anesthesia and Perioperative Care of the Combat Casualty, Vol 1. Textbook of Military Medicine. Washington, DC: Office of The Surgeon General at TMM Publications; 1995

[6] Bellamy RF, Zajtchuk R, Buescher TM, et al. Part I. Warfare, Weaponry, and the Casualty: Conventional Warfare: Ballistic, Blast, and Burn Injuries, Vol 5. Textbook of Military Medicine. Washington, DC: Office of the Surgeon General at TMM Publications; 1991

[7] Rotondo MF, Schwab CW, McGonigal MD, et al. "Damage control": An approach for improved survival in exsanguinating penetrating abdominal injury. The Journal of Trauma. 1993;**35**:375-382, discussion 382-373

[8] Satava RM. Robotic surgery: From past to future: A personal journey. The Surgical Clinics of North America. 2003;**83**:1491-1500

[9] Aaarts J, Nieboer T, Johnson N, et al. Surgical approach to hysterectomy for benign gynecological disease. Cochrane Database of Systematic Reviews. 2012;**12** Art No: CD003677

[10] Diaz-Arrastia C, Jurnalov C, Gomez G, Townsend C. Jr laparoscopic hysterectomy using a computer-enhanced surgical robot. Surgical Endoscopy. 2002;**16**:1271-1273

[11] Edward LF. The History of Robotic-Assisted Surgery. 2021. 978-3-030-53594-0

[12] Sergiu D, Laparoscopica C. Editia a doua. Editura Paralela. 2022;**45**:65-74

[13] Querleu D, Cibula D, Abu-Rustum NR. 2017 update on the Querleau-Morrow classification of radical hysterectomy. Annals of Surgical Oncology. 2017;**24**(11):3406-3412

[14] Ramirez PT, Frumovitz M, Pareja R, Lopez A, Vieira M, Ribeiro R, et al. Minimally invasive versus radical abdominal hysterectomy for cervical cancer. The New England Journal of Medicine. 2018;**379**(20):1895-1904

[15] Cibula D, Potter R, Planchamp F, et al. The European Society of Gynecological Oncology/ European Society of Pathology guidelines for the management of patients with cervical cancer. International Journal of Gynecological Cancer. 2018;**28**:641-655

[16] National Comprehensive Cancer Network. NCCN clinical practice

guidelines in oncology: cervical cancer (version I.2018). 2017. Availble from: http://oncolife.com.ua/doc/nccn/Cervical_Cancer.pdf

[17] Tran AQ, Sullivan SA, Gehrig PA, Soper JT, Boggess JF, Kim KH. Robotic radical parametrectomy with upper vaginectomy and pelvic lymphadenectomy in patients with occult cervical carcinoma after extra fascial hysterectomy. Journal of Minimally Invasive Gynecology. 2017;**24**(5):757-763

[18] Querleu D, Morrow CP. Classification of radical hysterectomy. The Lancet Oncology. 2008;**9**(3):297-300

[19] Chapron CM, Pierre F, Lacroix S, Querleu D, Lansac J, Dubuisson J-B. Major vascular injuries during gynecologic laparoscopy. Journal of the American College of Surgeons. 1997a;**185**:461-465

[20] Wisner KPA, Gupta S, Ahmad S, Holloway RW. Indications and techniques for robotic pelvic and Para-aortic lymphadenectomy in gynecologic oncology. Journal of Surgical Oncology. 2015;**112**(7):782-789

[21] Sharma C, Deutsch I, Lewin SN, et al. Lymphadenectomy influences the utilization of adjuvant radiation treatment for endometrial cancer. American Journal of Obstetrics and Gynecology. 2011;**205**(6):562-569

[22] Cibula D, Abu-Rustum NR. Pelvic lymphadenectomy in cervical cancer-surgical anatomy and proposal for the new classification system. Gynecologic Oncology. 2010 Jan;**116**(1):33-37

[23] Cusimano MC, Vicus D, Pulman K, Maganti M, Bernardini MQ, Bouchard-Fortier G, et al. Assessment of sentinel lymph node biopsy vs. lymphadenectomy for intermediate and high-grade endometrial cancer staging. JAMA Surgery. 2021;**156**(2):157-164

[24] Cormier B, Rozenholc AT, Gotlieb W, Plante M, Giede C, Communities of Practice (CoP) Group of Society of Gynecologic Oncology of Canada (GOC). Sentinel lymph node procedure in endometrial cancer: A systematic review and proposal for standardization of future research. Gynecologic Oncology. 2015;**138**(2):478-485

[25] Bodurtha SAJ, Fader AN, Tanner EJ. Sentinel lymph node assessment in endometrial cancer: A systematic review and meta-analysis. American Journal of Obstetrics and Gynecology. 2017;**216**(5):459-476

[26] Rossi EC, Kowalski LD, Scalici J, Cantrell L, Schuler K, Hanna RK, et al. A comparison of sentinel lymph node biopsy to lymphadenectomy for endometrial cancer staging (FIRES trial): A multicentre, prospective, cohort study. The Lancet Oncology. 2017;**18**(3):384-392

[27] Ngan TYT, Zakhari A, Czuzoj-Shulman N, Tulandi T, Abenheim HA. Laparoscopic and robotic-assisted hysterectomy for uterine leiomyomas: A comparison of complications and costs. Journal of Obstetrics and Gynaecology Canada. 2018 Apr;**40**(4):432-439

[28] Behbehani S, Delara R, Yi J, Kunze K, Suarez-Salvador E, Wasson M. Predictors of postoperative urinary retention in outpatient minimally invasive hysterectomy. Journal of Minimally Invasive Gynecology. 2020;**27**(3):681-686

[29] Kaye AD, Vadivelu N, Ahuja N, et al. Anesthetic considerations in robotic-assisted gynecologic surgery. The Ochsner Journal. 2013;**13**:517-524

[30] Iavazzo C, Gkegkes ID. Robotically assisted hysterectomy in obese patients: A systematic review. Archives of Gynecology and Obstetrics. 2016;**293**(6):1169-1183

[31] Liu CY, Reich H. Complications of total laparoscopic hysterectomy in 518 cases. Gynaecological Endoscopy. 1994;**3**:203-208

[32] Catanzarite T, Saha S, Pilecki MA, et al. The longer operative time during benign laparoscopic and robotic hysterectomy is associated with increased 30-day perioperative complications. Journal of Minimally Invasive Gynecology. 2015;**22**:1049-1058

[33] Marra AR, Puig-Asensio M, Edmond MB, Schweizer ML, Bender D. Infectious complications of laparoscopic and robotic hysterectomy: A systematic literature review and meta-analysis. International Journal of Gynecological Cancer. 2019;**29**(3):518-530

[34] Marret H, Harchaoui Y, Chapron C, Lansac J, Pierre F. Trocar injuries during laparoscopic gynecological surgery. Report from the French Society of Gynaecological Laparoscopy. Gynaecological Endoscopy. 1998;7:235-241

[35] Mencagalia L, Minelli L, Wattiez A. Manual of Gynecological Laparoscopic Surgery. 2nd ed. 2013. 978-3-89756-405-3

[36] Gorchev G, Kornovski IA. Anatomical and surgical meaning of the bladder during the performance of radical hysterectomy. Akusherstvo i Ginekologiia. 2006;**45**:24-27

[37] Hwang JH, Kim BW, Kim SR, Kim JH. Robotic radical hysterectomy is not superior to radical laparoscopic hysterectomy in perioperative urologic complications: A meta-analysis of 23 studies. Journal of Minimally Invasive Gynecology. 2020;**27**(1):38-47